AWAKEN & BECOME A TREE OF LIFE

Always Be Cleansing

Christine Maxwell
Cara Marie Ringland

**Awaken & Become
A Tree of Life**

Always Be Cleansing

**Christine Maxwell
Cara Marie Ringland**

All rights reserved. No part of this book may be reproduced or transmitted in any form or by any means without written permission from the author.

Int. Copyright © 2024 No. **CI- 28071313537**
ISBN: **978-1-7361998-2-4**

Printed in the U.S.A. by

CHRISTINE MAXWELL Group LLC

TABLE OF CONTENTS

Disclaimer: 5

In Loving Memory: 7

Acknowledgments: 10

Foreword: 14

Introduction To The Study of Iridology: 19

Meet The Father of Iridology: 21

Chapter 1: Health Is the Greatest Wealth 27

Chapter 2: The Theory and Practice of Alkaline Cleansing 41

Chapter 3: The Genetic Role of Eye Color 70

Chapter 4: Exploring Digestion and Enzyme Function 88

Chapter 5: Nutrition Guidelines to Support Enzyme Function 95

Chapter 6: Hydration Standards for Wellness 105

Chapter 7: Additional Practices to Create A "New Start" 118

Chapter 8: Setting The Stage for Success 139

Bonus: 149

Resources: 162

Affirmations/Prayer: 166

Contacts: 170

DISCLAIMER

Christine Maxwell and Cara Marie Ringland make no medical claims. Information provided in this book is for educational purposes and is not intended to diagnose, prescribe, or substitute for medical care. The FDA and AMA regulate the practice of medicine. Claims about the impact of vitamins, herbs, etc., are unlawful. Practicing health does not require a license. A Traditional Naturopath complements medical care without replacing it, offering information to promote vibrant health.

CAUTION

This program is not a cure but a method to cleanse the bowel and restore regular habits, leading to a clean, healthy body. While rarely conflicting with other therapies, it's advisable to discuss it with a doctor, especially if under medical care. These suggestions do not replace professional health care. For the seriously ill or elderly, modify under a doctor's advice. The book is comprehensive, but questions are welcome. For severe bowel issues, doctor supervision is imperative.

We strongly urge all participants to obtain medical blood work and physical examinations, particularly for those who do not already possess these records. This will empower individuals with valuable health information.

IN LOVING MEMORY

In honor and memory of Alfredo Bowman, born in Honduras in 1933, renowned globally as Dr. Sebi, a healer revered by countless individuals for his remarkable treatments of various diseases. I express heartfelt gratitude to him for instilling in me the significance of comprehending our bodies and the significance of alkaline electrical foods. Your wisdom and knowledge have indelibly altered the course of my life. I am forever transformed by the wealth of insights you imparted. I am committed to perpetuating your legacy by generously sharing the invaluable treasures I gained from you with all those providentially crossing my path. May you rest in peace as your work continues in the lives of others.

Christine Maxwell

DEDICATION

This book is a tribute to Dr. Carol Deanna Geeck. Her vibrant spirit, thirst for life, and tenacity led her to intern with Dr. Bernard Jensen. Carol trained me in the same manner. Carol was born on March 24, 1940, and departed peacefully on May 30, 2022, leaving her legacy in my care.

I also dedicate this to my mother, Kim Marie Ringland, born April 26,1955. She devoted her life to "Intentional Living," staying close to nature. She taught me how to read, write, and tend to plants and animals. Her expertise as a Master Herbalist became renowned wherever she lived. Her zest for living and her generous nature made her unforgettable to those who met her. On May 28, 2022, she left this world.

Lastly, I honor my grandfather, Dr. Otto Hakon Ravenholt, who was born May 17,1927. He served as the coroner and Health Officer of Las Vegas, Nevada, in 1962, serving 36 years. He was indeed a remarkable man named "The Good Doctor" by the people of Las Vegas and dubbed the "High

Priest of Health" in the state of Nevada. It is dear to my heart to fulfill my promise to him to publish. He departed on March 18, 2012.

Cara Marie Ringland

ACKNOWLEDGEMENTS

Firstly, I attribute all the Glory to God for profoundly inspiring me with His divine love, an eternal force that continually reshapes my life with each passing day. This love, permeating through me, stands poised to catalyze the transformation of others.

To Brian & Anna Marie Clement of the Hippocrates Health Institute, I extend my deepest gratitude for your invaluable teachings and the profound experiences that have transformed my life. Your guidance and wisdom have been instrumental in shaping my understanding of health, wellness, mind, soul, and emotions. I am dedicated to perpetuating your teachings, committed to the noble cause of changing the world, one individual at a time, just as you have shown and inspired me to do.

Heartfelt gratitude extends to Prophetess Gwendolyn Bradley, whose prophetic vision foresaw Cara and me collaborating on a book. Your prayers are deeply appreciated and cherished.

Acknowledgement and heartfelt appreciation are extended to Dr. Ellen Jensen, my esteemed Iridology Professor, whose gentle yet powerful and loving demeanor imparted profound lessons on the healing potential of this remarkable tool in a non-invasive manner. Your inspiring vision of me assisting community leaders will forever resonate within me, serving as a guiding light and a lasting source of motivation.

Christine Maxwell

CREDITS

I am grateful beyond measure for the breath of life and the power of God's love to lead me on this journey. Faith has truly proven to carry me through time and again. I reverently acknowledge the miracles prayer has gifted to my life.

Working with Christine Maxwell on this assignment, prophesied by Prophetess Gwendolyn Bradley, is a great honor. Christine's experienced background, alongside her grace, wisdom, and patience, is a guiding light.

I offer gratitude to Dr. Ellen Tart-Jensen for instructing me in the techniques of Iris Analysis. Iridology has been the backbone of my adult life as a parent and professional.

Ed Geeck has become one of my dearest friends and a tremendous supporter of this endeavor. Sharing this achievement with him is rich and endearing. I sincerely thank my children, Chloe and Matthew Young, for their unconditional love. I extend gratitude to Ryan Young for being a consistent friend over all the years. I appreciate my father, Craig Ringland, for his loving presence, uncanny words of wisdom, and love. I thank my sister, Kristine Ringland, for growing up beside me. I offer gratitude to Nevada City, California, for fostering a beautiful life.

Cara Marie Ringland

FOREWORD

It is with great pleasure that I write the foreword to this life-changing book, Awaken & Become A Tree of Life, Always Be Cleansing. The information in this book is vital, especially at this time in the United States and throughout the world, when cancer, heart disease, and diabetes are taking the lives of too many people and causing heartache for all those family members left behind. Most people have no clue that their lifestyle and the way they eat is causing most of their health problems. They are becoming weary of taking medications that simply mask the symptoms but have no understanding of the fundamental basics of how to restore their health and live happy lives. I have spent over 40 years in the field of iridology, nutrition, and naturopathy and have had the opportunity to study with some of the best natural healers in the world. Some of my greatest knowledge and understanding of the healing laws of God and nature came from my extensive training for five years with Dr. Bernard Jensen at the Hidden Valley Health Ranch in California.

Bernard Jensen became ill from tuberculosis as a young man and was able to finally heal through nutrition and natural therapies after no medicine had helped him. He became a pioneer for sixty years, teaching iridology, good nutrition, and colon cleansing in over fifty countries.

With his instruction, I learned the fundamental keys for vibrant health and long life through cleansing the body, drinking pure water, exercise, having happy thoughts, and getting the nutrients we need in whole, fresh, natural foods grown in rich organic soil containing all the 90 essential elements needed for health.

People came to see Dr. Bernard Jensen from all over the world and miracles occurred. Since that time, I have traveled and lectured worldwide on the ways and means to achieve radiant health, and I have maintained a busy practice of coaching thousands of people who were able to bring bodies back into balance.

The authors of this wonderful book, Cara Ringland and Christine Maxwell, studied with me extensively, and they also studied with the great Dr. Carol Geeck, Dr. Sebi, and Drs. Brian and Anna Marie Clement, and others. Together, they have joined forces to help make a difference in this world and have shared their cumulative knowledge here. Both ladies endured severe health concerns, have turned their lives around, and now have great health.

This is a beautiful book, well-written step-by-step, very clear, and easy to understand. It will give you all the important information you need to prevent illness or restore your body to vibrant health. In this book, you will learn about iridology and how the eyes, which are intricately connected to the nerves and all the organs, glands, and tissues, can show areas of the body that are inherently strong and areas that need extra care. Even the color of the eyes tells a great deal about genetics and guides us to know which foods are best suited to that genetic type. You will learn the intrinsic value of keeping the lymph fluid alkaline, which will help prevent arthritis and other serious dis-ease.

Many people are living "life on the go," grabbing fast foods daily, and as is stated here, "leveraging every available tool is vital when embarking on new ventures." You will learn how important pure water, exercise, eating healthy foods, fasting, prayer, and stillness can be to keep your mind calm and clear. A calm, clear mind will give you the needed desire to take care of your beautiful body temple so that you can become a "tree of life" and fulfill your purpose here on earth, feeling well and joyful.

In this informative health manual that will become your best friend, you can look up various ailments, therapies, and recipes to guide you as you embark on your health journey. Cleansing mystery out of cleansing gives clear directions on making a "New Start" in your lives, covering all you need to know about nutrition, exercise, water, sunshine, temperance, air, rest, and trust in Divine Power.

I highly recommend this book for all mothers, fathers, teachers, health care professionals, and lay people who want to improve their own health or their children's health. You will enjoy each great health tool provided and feel healthier each day that you apply these principles for a long and meaningful life. Enjoy!

Ellen Tart Jensen
Health is Your Birthright
Techniques in Iris Analysis

INTRODUCTION TO THE STUDY OF IRIDOLOGY
by Cara

Eyes are often deemed the windows to the soul, revealing insights into one's health. Iridology, dating back to the 1800s, interprets colors, textures, and patterns in the iris to identify underlying inflammation causes. Reflex charts, akin to hand and foot reflexology maps, connect nerve endings to organs. The iris, formed during embryonic development, reflects genetic strengths, weaknesses, and personality traits.

Iridology brings awareness to alkaline balance and elimination, correlating to how genetic constitutions often absorb nutrition and eliminate waste. Tissue vitality diminishes with poor nutrient absorption and acidic waste accumulation, setting the stage for health issues.

Iridologists evaluate tissue integrity for signs of metabolic activity, helping identify overactive or stagnant tissues.

Understanding genetic inheritances empowers individuals to support their overall well-being. Adopting a lifestyle focused on alkalizing and daily waste elimination enhances nutrient absorption. Genetic factors, combined with nutrition, environment, lifestyle, exposure to chemicals, stress, and age, contribute to overall health. Epigenetics explores improving genetics through diet and lifestyle for prevention, with Iridology offering keys to restoring wellness in body, mind, and spirit.

MEET THE FATHER OF IRIDOLOGY

"Good health allows the person to become the individual he wants to be and to obtain the highest goals in life. Of all the earthly treasures, vibrant health is the most precious."

Dr. Bernard Jensen

Meet Dr. Bernard Jensen, the Father of Modern Iridology, who dedicated his life to the field. Graduating as a Chiropractor in 1929, he earned a diploma in Iris Analysis in 1932. Jensen's extensive research as a Naturopath and his technological contributions, such as the first eye photography camera, laid the foundation for modern Iridology.

He traveled to over 50 countries to study the lifestyles of the different cultures in an effort to understand the principles of longevity. After visiting many of Europe's spas and natural health sanitariums, he brought many of these ideas back to development at the Hidden Valley Health Ranch in 1955, located in Escondido, California. It was a place for his patients and guests to come and learn how to cleanse and live a healthy life.

Dr. Jensen concluded that the long-lived people live a simple life in a moderate temperature, eat unprocessed foods, no fried foods, little meat, live a serene, contented life, maintain good posture, and consistently live close to the black soil.

Dr. Jensen believed humanity needs a simple formula for living successfully, healthfully, and peacefully. He combined physical, mental, and spiritual elements in teaching people how to live rich and fulfilling lives.

In the late 1980s, Carol Geeck, inspired by Jensen, immersed herself in Iridology. Becoming Jensen's intern, she met Dr. Ellen Tart at the Hidden Valley Health Ranch, where they formed a close relationship. Both women and other original students established the IIPA (International Iridology Practitioner's Association) organization to standardize global education and conduct scientific research in Iridology.

Dr. Ellen Tart-Jensen married Art Jensen, becoming his daughter-in-law, and took up the mantle where the beloved Bernard left off. Serving as the President of IIPA, founder of "My Infinite Iris," and Director of Bernard Jensen International, she is recognized as one of the world's leading Iridologists. If Jensen is the Father of Modern Iridology, Ellen and Carol are his beloved daughters, passing the tradition to the next generation—Cara Marie Ringland and Christine Maxwell. The family's Iridology legacy continues, imparting wisdom for generations to come.

This iridology chart, the inaugural standardized version, is a result of Dr. Ellen Jensen's research and holds international recognition.

Fig. 1

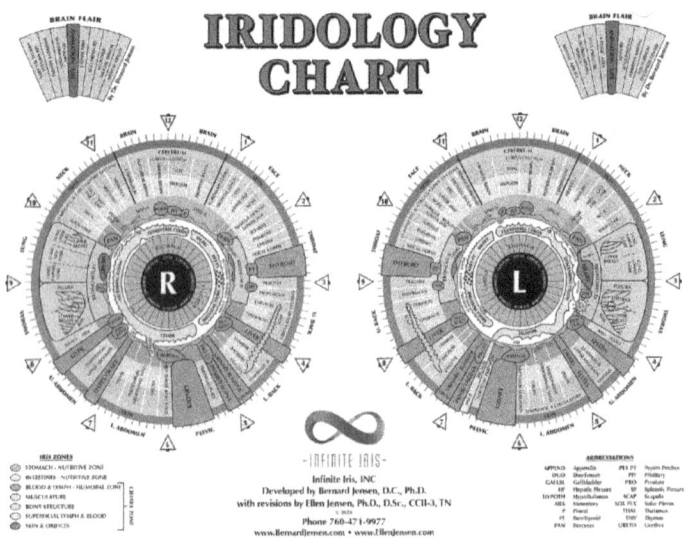

For consultations, please email us at
Eye.readologycc@gmail.com

CAPTURE A PHOTO OF YOUR EYE USING A MIRROR AND YOUR SMARTPHONE, AND USE THE CHART ON THE PREVIOUS PAGE TO DO SELF ASSESSMENT.

1. Stand in front of a clean bathroom mirror with room lights on.
2. Open your smartphone's photo app and use the back camera.
3. In photo mode, turn on the flash, set 2-2.5x zoom, and hold the phone in the hand corresponding to the eye you're photographing.
4. Point the camera at your eye, ensuring the display faces the mirror.
5. Turn the phone horizontally, placing your finger on the volume button.
6. Align the eye in the mirror reflection to the center of the display and fill the frame.
7. Maintain about a 4-inch distance between the camera lens and your eye.
8. Take a focused picture by pressing the volume button or the on-screen button.

9. Repeat for the other eye, ensuring both eyes are photographed separately.
10. Avoid obstructions and shadows on the eye; center the eye in the picture.
11. If needed, ask a family member or friend to assist, using 2-2.5x zoom and flash about 4 inches away.
12. Ensure your phone's camera is clean and not too close to the eye to prevent blurry images.

CHAPTER 1
HEALTH IS THE GREATEST WEALTH

"The road to health is the one that begins with an understanding and commitment to cleanse and detoxify the body, to restore balance, peace, and harmony. We must be willing to rise above selfish habits, realizing that the path of cleansing has implications for the intellect, emotions, and spirit. We need to accept our personal responsibility on this path." - Dr. Bernard Jensen

The leaves of the trees are for the healing of the nation. Revelation 22:2

Dr. Bernard Jensen emphasized the topics below inspired by his book "Tissue Cleansing Through Bowel Management."

PROPER LIVING HABITS

Living a healthy life should render concerns about bowel function unnecessary. Unfortunately, many of us fail to adopt proper habits. Our diets lack nutrition. We neglect exercise, fresh air, and sunshine. Expecting optimal bowel function becomes unrealistic with so much amiss in our routines.

Today's disease statistics reflect these shortcomings. Medical attention is predominantly aimed at treating issues stemming from poor lifestyle choices.

These detrimental habits stem from modern civilization and inherited lifestyles. Despite our perception of progress, it's evident that many modern advancements compromise our health. It's imperative to rectify this discrepancy. Doctors focus primarily on treating ailments, neglecting the crucial role of teaching proper living practices. It's time for a shift to educate people on how to live healthily.

AN OUNCE OF EDUCATION IS WORTH A POUND OF CURE

Understanding how to achieve and maintain good health is crucial. Individuals vary in their comprehension and approach to wellness, requiring tailored guidance. Some prioritize spending exorbitantly on treatments and products. However, true health cannot be bought; it must be earned through effort and dedication.

Many current treatments fail to impart the knowledge of proper self-care, leaving patients unchanged in their awareness. The path to improved health remains elusive without elevating one's mental attitude and consciousness.

CLEANSING & DETOXIFICATION

Cleansing and detoxification remain an often-overlooked aspect within the realm of healing despite its crucial significance acknowledged by health professionals. A sick body invariably indicates an acidic body, where toxic acids result from natural cell breakdown and additional assimilation of toxins from our surroundings—be it the air we breathe, the food we consume, chemicals on our skin, or other environmental factors. When the body efficiently expels these toxins, there's no cause for concern. However, trouble arises when the body either absorbs toxins faster than it eliminates them or experiences underactive elimination. The accumulation of toxins and acids within the body is known to create the necessary groundwork for the onset of diseases.

The "Always Be Cleansing" phrase, introduced by Christine, is an alkalizing mindset. It teaches how to assist the body with daily elimination while reducing exposure to known toxins and consuming high-nutrient alkaline foods.

PROPER ELIMINATION & BOWEL HEALTH

Proper elimination is paramount among the myriad of processes crucial for optimal health. When evaluating bodily systems, it becomes evident that effective bowel management holds a pivotal role. Health issues predominantly stem from the bowel compared to other body parts. A clean bowel is essential for the body's well-being.

The cleanliness of various tissues—be it the kidneys, stomach, or even the brain—is contingent upon the condition of the bowel.

Addressing bowel health is crucial for overall well-being, as it plays a pivotal role in the body's cleansing process. Recognizing that a healthy bowel contributes to healthy blood and healthier cells throughout the body underscores the importance of thorough bowel cleansing. While discussing bowel health might be considered socially uncomfortable, it is an essential aspect of maintaining overall health, and open dialogue is necessary to provide the support many individuals may need in this regard.

MENTAL WELL-BEING

"Should the body use the mind before the court judicature for damages, it would be found that the mind had been a ruinous tenant to its landlord."
-Essays of Plutarch

Addressing the intertwined realms of physical and mental imbalances is crucial. The mind's influence can induce tension, leading to contractions in the bowel wall. One might attribute the onset of colitis to mental origins. Stress and nerve-induced responses can trigger bowel inflammation. Emotional distress, including financial worries, often correlates with irregular bowel movements, while freedom from such stressors can significantly improve bowel function. Positive factors like routine and relaxation can foster healthier bowel movements.

Understanding how to achieve and maintain good health is crucial. Individuals vary in their comprehension and approach to wellness, requiring tailored guidance. Proper health cannot be bought; it must be earned through effort and dedication. Many current treatments fail to impart knowledge, leaving patients unchanged in their awareness. The path to improved health remains elusive without elevating one's mental attitude and consciousness.

The emphasis lies in caring for the bowel rather than relying solely on drugs, supplements, or injections. While each method may offer some improvement, genuine rectification demands a comprehensive understanding of proper living. It's not just about food or diet; it extends to harmonious relationships and lifestyle choices. Achieving optimal bowel function necessitates more than isolated treatments—it requires embracing a wholesome way of life.

Often, the issue doesn't solely reside within an individual; it may stem from poor interpersonal relationships, negative influences, trauma, and toxic environments or behaviors.

Understanding the intricate link between mental and physical health is fundamental in fostering a balanced and harmonious life, positively influencing the functionality of our bodily systems, including the bowel.

"The bowel-wise person is the one who is armed with good knowledge, practices discrimination in his eating habits, and walks the path of the higher life. His days are blessed with health, vitality, optimism, and the fulfillment of life's goals. He is a blessing and source of inspiration to family and associates. His cheerful disposition comes from having a vital, toxin-free body made possible by a loved and well-cared-for bowel's efficient, regular, and cleansing action. Every person who desires the higher things in life must be aware of proper bowel management, what it is, how it works, and what is required.

In doing so, you will discover many secrets of life, develop a positive attitude toward yourself, and become the master of body function."

From the book "Mysterious Catalytic Foods," written by Brown Landone

CARA'S PATH TO IRIDOLOGY

Raised in a family dedicated to natural health, my upbringing involved off-grid, country living in Northern Idaho with "Back to Land" parents. My mother studied to be a Master Herbalist and organic farmer who chose to homeschool my sister and me while guiding us in the art of sustainable living, herbalism, and animal care.

My father's work in elderly care and my grandfather's extraordinary medical expertise profoundly influenced my fascination with preventative health.

Following personal encounters with severe health issues for my sister and me, my quest for natural alternatives to chemical medicine led me to Dr. Carol Geeck, a Naturopath and Iridologist, in the year 2000. Our immediate connection initiated a mentor-student relationship wherein Dr. Geeck employed me after I received my Iridology instruction under Dr. Ellen Tart-Jensen. My subsequent 3-year internship at Lifestyle Transformation Health and Research Clinic exposed me to the miracles of ancient and modern advances in natural healing and detoxification practices.

Carol expanded her studies to include Live Blood Cell Analysis, Allergy Testing, Clinical Aromatherapy, Emotional Release, and much more. As a leading Naturopath, she served to help build The Young Life Research Clinic in Utah and worked at The Tree of Life Institute in Arizona. Dr. Geeck's clinical approach carefully instructed me to preserve the wisdom she gathered in her lifetime.

The practices detailed in this book that emphasize alkalizing, cleansing, and hydrotherapy stem primarily from the teachings of Dr. Bernard Jensen. These traditions were the foundation of my internship with Dr. Geeck and my training with Dr. Tart-Jensen. Ellen's contributions to IIPA, the International Iridology Practitioner's Association, continue to standardize Iridology's research, curriculum, and application worldwide.

Meeting Christine Maxwell during an Iridology class with our esteemed instructor has been a profound blessing. To author this book together is a great honor. We both passionately advocate for returning to nature and recognizing food as our primary medicine. Embracing the ethos of "Always Be Cleansing," a term introduced to me by Christine, promotes preventive wellness in the face of modern challenges such as weakened genetics, increased pollution, and inadequate nutrition. This book serves as a vessel for sharing this invaluable wisdom. May these words serve as a beacon for those desiring to live in harmony with the principles of natural health, embodying the spirit of A Tree of Life.

CHRISTINE'S JOURNEY TO IRIDOLOGY AS A CERTIFIED HEALTH EDUCATOR & COACH

In my quest for health and well-being, I came upon Iridology, or perhaps it found me. During my journey to become a certified health educator at the Hippocrates Health Institute, I encountered various health modalities, and Iridology struck a deep chord within me. This fascination led me to embark on the path of becoming an Iridologist.

My exploration into Iridology introduced me to Dr. Ellen Jensen, a teacher who followed the teachings of Bernard Jensen, often regarded as the Father of Iridology. Through my studies, I crossed paths with remarkable individuals. I met Cara Ringland while attending a class taught by Dr. Ellen Jensen in California. Our shared passion for promoting health and wellness through diverse modalities brought us together to write this book. We hope to help others utilize Iridology as this amazing tool to map a way to divine health and wholeness.

I have developed a genuine affinity for Iridology due to its noninvasive approach to analyzing our genetic strengths and weaknesses. By examining the iris, the area around the pupil, and the sclera of the eye, we can gain valuable insights into our health conditions. We aim to extend this knowledge to others, helping them make informed decisions about their diets, nutrient intake, cleansing routines, exercise, and more to live healthier lives.

I have discovered that the principle encapsulated in the phrase "ABC," signifying Always Be Cleansing - resonates profoundly in my quest for holistic well-being encompassing body, soul, and spirit. Sharing this mantra with my clients, friends, and family is a practice I ardently maintain, aspiring for its universal benefit and aid to all. This phrase is in the subtitle and will be used throughout this book.

Dr. Jensen eloquently emphasizes the inseparable connection between Iridology and Nutrition, stating, "Iridology and Nutrition are like twins. They cannot be separated." In the pages of this book, we will guide you through the fundamental techniques of Iridology and alkaline cleansing, hoping that you will also come to appreciate and harness the incredible potential benefits this modality offers.

REFLECTIONS

CHAPTER 2
THE THEORY AND PRACTICE OF ALKALINE CLEANSING

"The human body has no place for acidity; the body is alkaline." ~ Dr. Sebi

*Along each bank of the river, every kind of fruit tree will grow; their leaves will not wither, nor will their fruit fail.
Ezekiel 47:12*

CHRISTINE'S INITIATION INTO AN ALKALINE CLEANSING LIFESTYLE

My personal healing journey led me to Dr. Sebi's wisdom, Alfredo Bowman, who emphasized the significance of alkaline electrical foods and understanding our bodies. This knowledge transformed my life, and I'm committed to preserving his legacy by sharing the valuable insights I gained. In our toxin-filled world, maintaining an alkaline state is vital for optimal health, although it's not always easy. Even the smallest steps in this direction can significantly affect our overall health and well-being.

Alkalinity and cleansing are inseparable companions on the path to health. Straying too far into acidity (pH below 6) can lead to inflammation, sickness, and disease. This book is designed to guide you in maintaining balance through proper nutrition and effective cleansing. Implementing its principles sets you on a path to wholeness.

Our bodies consist of millions of living cells, which are crucial to our overall health. When these cells cannot function properly, they can produce unhealthy cells, contributing to illness. Non-hybrid, unaltered foods with intact genetic integrity, such as seeded fruits, are essential for optimal health.

The connection between electrical, alkaline foods and our well-being is deeply rooted in nature and history. Dr. Sebi emphasized the pivotal role of iron in our health, highlighting it as one of the most crucial minerals. According to his teachings, iron is a vital nourishment for the brain, playing a fundamental role in our overall well-being.

He observed that individuals grappling with illness often exhibited signs of anemia, underlining the significance of iron deficiency in various health issues. Furthermore, Dr. Sebi pointed out that iron acts as a chief orchestrator in the body, attracting and influencing the absorption of other essential minerals.

He stressed that insufficient iron intake renders one vulnerable to various diseases. Notably, he illuminated the unique characteristic of iron being the sole magnetic mineral on the planet, illustrating its unparalleled significance.

In his teachings, Dr. Sebi enlightened us about the extensive presence of minerals in the natural world, noting that there are 102 minerals in all naturally occurring entities. He vividly illustrated this by suggesting that even the analysis of clouds in a laboratory would reveal the presence of these 102 minerals.

He further exemplified this concept by drawing attention to sea salt, highlighting that it contains the full spectrum of these 102 minerals, mirroring the composition found in the human body. According to his teachings, this comprehensive mineral profile is intrinsic to maintaining our health and vitality.

In various teachings, the correlation between oxygen deprivation and the onset of diseases is underscored. The body's gradual erosion, caused by an acidic environment and mucus buildup, is believed to obstruct the efficient transportation and utilization of oxygen. This deprivation is seen as a pivotal factor contributing to the development and progression of numerous health issues.

Dr. Sebi and others have stressed the significance of creating and maintaining an alkaline environment in the body, highlighting its pivotal role in ensuring proper oxygenation.

They advocated for measures to counteract acidity and mucus accumulation, emphasizing their detrimental impact on oxygen levels. Addressing these factors aims to support the body in achieving and sustaining optimal health through enhanced oxygenation and alkalinity.

Cleansing is beneficial and necessary due to our deviation from our original design. ***"Always Be Cleansing" (ABC)*** should be our motto. This book focuses on the daily practices of alkalizing and cleansing our bodies, addressing common issues like constipation, a significant impediment to health. Applying the techniques outlined in this book can make the cleansing process more manageable and less daunting, ultimately safeguarding your well-being.

Poem - Author Unknown

Starch and blood will cause a flood that floods the brain that brings the pain that makes her blame.

I was fortunate to dig deeper into the realm of cleansing during my time at the Hippocrates Health Institute situated in West Palm, Florida. Founded by the co-founders Brian and Anna Marie Clements, whose philosophy was originally instilled by Ann Wigmore, their teachings also permeate the essence of this enlightening book. Immersed in a comprehensive 12-week study in 2019, I absorbed invaluable insights centered not solely on physical cleansing protocols but also on fostering a profound connection with an expression of overall well-being – encompassing the realms of the physical, mental, emotional, and spiritual aspects. This immersion was rooted in a holistic living foods lifestyle, emphasizing the pivotal role that knowledge, skills, and experiential learning play in our healing and overall health.

The transformative journey I embarked upon was indeed profound, and I remain immensely grateful for the profound changes it ushered into my life. The process of cleansing, which entailed various modalities such as infrared saunas, raw and living foods, green juice, fasting, sprouts, wheatgrass, chlorella, colonics, hydrotherapy, exercise, and ample rest, among others, all coalesced harmoniously to facilitate an alkaline cleansing vital for revitalization and restoration.

Hippocrates believes the first step in the healing process is to remove as many toxins from the body as possible to allow the organs and immune system to operate most efficiently. These toxins are most often embedded in the body's cell structure, so we must rebuild the body to introduce healthy cells to regenerate health, which means initiating a detoxification regimen. They believe everyone should consider undergoing detoxification as a process for maintaining health. How, one may ask. A juice fast one day a week would be helpful. Exercise, colon cleansing, and eating pure, natural, organic food also help. Having a detox strategy for yourself and those you love is a survival mechanism that can help maintain good health and maybe even prevent premature death.

4 TIPS FROM HIPPOCRATES FOR CLEANSING

- If you are constipated, colon cleansing should be the first step.
- Fasting might be the next step if you have poor digestion or a cold.
- Exercise that works up a sweat can effectively remove some toxins from the body via perspiration.
- Chlorella is at the top of the detox list. It is the most effective of the green algae in taking out heavy metals and radiation from the body, as it has a mineral complex that magnetizes toxins and acts as a sponge to soak them up.

THE ROLE OF COLON HYDROTHERAPY
Hippocrates view

They use enemas and colonic irrigation treatment utilizing wheatgrass or algae implants. During decades of research, they found that this practice helps to restore the electrolyte and mineral balance in the colon while cleansing the system of toxins. Cleansing the colon with water dates from ancient times, and some western hospitals continued the practice until the 1940s.

THE ROLE OF LYMPHATIC DRAINAGE MASSAGE

This body-massage technique assists the flow of lymph along its normal glandular routes. The goal is to reduce congestion and the retention of wastes and strengthen the immune system.

THE ROLE OF FAR-INFRARED SAUNAS

A relatively recent but essential component of our detox program involves using far-infrared saunas, which produce high energy as opposed to the high heat of conventional saunas. Far-infrared energy safely penetrates at least three inches into body tissues to help release chemical toxins that regular saunas fail to reach and excrete. Sweating out toxins has a rich historical tradition.

Whether it was sweat lodges in North American Indigenous cultures, the saunas popularized in Nordic cultures, or Turkish steam baths, people have long understood the benefits of detoxifying the body for both physical and spiritual purposes.

THE ROLE OF PHYSICAL EXERCISE

Vigorous physical activity is one of the human body's greatest allies in the fight against environmental toxicity. When we exercise, our lymphatic and respiratory systems, which include the lungs and the skin (our largest body organ), release some of the chemicals we absorb daily, which our body stores. Our bloodstream carries nutrients extracted from the food we eat to every cell in our body. Exercise facilitates the journey of these nutrients while generating enormous amounts of oxygen in the bloodstream. This highly oxygenated blood helps burn the nutrients that constitute our fuel more readily. Exercise quite literally nourishes our cells. Our bloodstream is also a sanitation department, clearing our systems of any residue that remains after the food fuel has been burned. Vigorous exercise helps the bloodstream to perform that role more efficiently. Finally, an unimpeded bloodstream keeps our veins and arteries open, inhibiting cholesterol accumulation.

Cara's path and mine share striking similarities, and we firmly believe that this recurring theme throughout this book underscores the crucial importance of alkaline cleansing and detoxification and their role in fostering healing and overall wellness.

CARA'S JOURNEY INTO THE REALM OF ALKALINE CLEANSING

At Lifestyle Transformation Health and Research Clinic, I learned a step-by-step systematic approach focusing on alkaline cleansing and daily self-care. I also studied advanced detoxification, known as "Tissue Cleansing Through Bowel Management," based on Dr. Bernard Jensen's methods. We drew wisdom from Dr. Stanley Burroughs with "The Master Cleanser" and applied the principles for healing and purification preserved in "The Essene Gospel of Peace" and "The Dead Sea Scrolls."

Alkalizing forms the foundation for good health, akin to priming a canvas for painting a masterpiece. "Cleansing" is defined in this book as daily "housekeeping" activities to support the natural elimination of metabolic wastes through the colon, kidneys, lungs, and skin - a vital practice.

Christine's introduction to me of the term ABC, "Always Be Cleansing," simply emphasizes the need to support our natural daily elimination processes. Like wiping the counter, it's best done daily.

"Detoxification" in this book refers to periodic deep cleaning, similar to cleaning a home after extended use. It's crucial to periodically "steam clean" the body's tissues to remove accumulated deposits of acids and toxins. "Fasting" refers to avoiding acid-forming foods and modern chemical toxins.

Maintaining a slightly alkaline pH balance of approximately 7.3 in the body is crucial for optimal cellular functions and for the body to transport oxygen and nutrients effectively.

The liver and pancreas play vital roles in managing blood pH balance by producing alkalizing bile and pancreatic juices to aid digestion.

Foods leave alkaline or acidic residues in the body based on mineral content. The body has strong disease resistance when the ratio of these residues is 80% alkaline to 20% acid. Acid-forming foods activate mucus production as an alkalizing agent, signaling over-acidity. Over activity = Over acidity.

The ability of the liver to filter the blood and distribute acids to be expelled through the kidneys, skin, colon, and lungs is essential to prevent imbalances. When the acids cannot be adequately eliminated, they deposit in the tissues, joints, vessels, and fluids.

Persistent acidity may lead to various cystic growths and degenerative health issues, highlighting the vital importance of alkalization.

The approach to incorporate alkaline cleansing as a lifestyle aligns with the concept of preventing and alleviating chronic conditions by addressing the body's pH balance. This holistic perspective is woven throughout the field of Iridology and provides invaluable insights for promoting overall health and well-being.

THE LINK BETWEEN THE TREE OF LIFE AND THE "ABC" PRINCIPLE: "ALWAYS BE CLEANSING."
by Cara

"Gray are all the theories, green is the tree of life." -
Goethe
The fruit of the righteous is a tree of life, and the one who is wise saves lives.
Proverbs 11:30

Drawing parallels between caring for trees and cultivating vibrant health in the human body is a compelling analogy. The concept of "As above, so below; as within so without" applies to both, emphasizing the importance of healthy roots in trees and intestinal villi in humans for absorbing nutrients. Healthy roots equal healthy fruits! Alkaline balance is vital in nutrient absorption, disease resistance, and overall well-being for both trees and humans.

Similarities in the effects of compact soil on trees and low-fiber diets on nutrient absorption highlight nutrition's impact on both species' health. The analogy extends to the significance of proper hydration, where the quality and quantity of water directly affect the well-being of trees and human tissues.

Exposure to chemicals and toxic substances has detrimental effects on trees and humans. The numerous consequences of overcrowded urban planting align with the challenges of sedentary living and lack of time in nature with sunshine and fresh air in human living environments. All life thrives with quality air, water, sunlight, and nutrition.

This image extends to reflect how pathogens and pests thrive in trees with weakened roots and acidic conditions. Similarly, fungal, viral, bacterial, or parasitic conditions can overpopulate human bodies under deficient or stressful circumstances. Genetic inheritances in trees and humans will likely manifest into degenerative diseases under physical or emotional stress.

The vision of vibrant trees in natural forests living in balance and producing abundant fruit resonates with the idea of individuals forming healthy, co-creative ecosystems and communities for wellness, prosperity, and purpose.

The call-to-action to "Always Be Cleansing" encapsulates the daily care standard for maintaining health and wellness in the urban world. This potent visual beautifully illustrates the interconnectedness of nature's principles and the well-being of trees and humans when cared for with harmonious conditions for their intended designs.

WHEN TO USE AN ALKALIZING TONIC

- When sickness has developed -for all acute and chronic conditions.
- When the digestive system needs a rest and a cleansing.
- When weight gain has become a problem.
- When better assimilation and building of body tissue is needed.
- When there is an overproduction of mucus.
- When pain and inflammation are present.
- When there are allergic reactions.

PURPOSE

- Dissolves toxins and congestion that have formed in the body.
- Cleanse the kidneys and the digestive system.
- Purifies the glands and cells throughout the entire body.
- Eliminates all waste and hardened material in the joints and muscles.

- Relieves pressure and irritation in the nerves, and blood vessels.

The esteemed physicians represented below offer these protocols as a quick method to alkalize the body. It is suggested to choose one or alternate between the two recipes according to one's preference.

THE MASTER CLEANSER BY STANLEY BURROUGHS

LEMONADE TONIC
2 TBSP Lemon or lime juice
1 tsp Blackstrap Molasses or Grade B Maple Syrup
1/4 tsp cayenne powder or 1 tsp ginger powder
12-16 ounces pure water

DR. JENSEN'S PROTOCOL FOR ALKALIZING

RAW APPLE CIDER VINEGAR TONIC

1 tsp Raw Apple Cider Vinegar

(Rice Vinegar for those with fungal infestations)

1 tsp honey

¼ tsp cinnamon powder or ginger powder

12-16 ounces of pure water

THE BENEFITS OF RAW APPLE CIDER VINEGAR

Antifungal and Antibacterial Effects:

Its properties make it effective against common fungal disorders and bacteria, including those responsible for staph infections, showcasing its antimicrobial qualities.

Kidney Stone Dissolution:

The acidic nature of raw apple cider vinegar may help decrease the size of kidney stones, aiding in their gradual breakdown. This can potentially facilitate their passage through the urinary tract, reducing the risk of stone formation.

Body Cleansing:

Regular consumption of raw apple cider vinegar may assist in flushing toxins from the body, contributing to reduced inflammation and pain.

Digestive Support:

The alkalizing effect of raw apple cider vinegar supports digestion and stimulates hydrochloric acid production.

Weight Loss Aid:

Raw Apple Cider Vinegar is known for its appetite-decreasing effect, promoting feelings of fullness, and reducing calorie intake. It can contribute to weight management by lowering blood sugar and insulin levels and promoting satiety. Combining it with honey in your daily diet may also help reduce belly fat and decrease blood triglycerides. It is known to be a diuretic that draws fluids and swelling from congested tissues.

THE HISTORY OF THE MASTER CLEANSER

"Alkalize or die." - Theodore Baroody

The lemonade diet, dating back to the early 1900s, as researched by Dr. Stanley Burroughs, has consistently demonstrated its healing and cleansing abilities. Lemons and limes, rich in minerals and vitamins, are available year-round, making this diet universally applicable.

Mucus disorders result from consuming mucus-forming foods. Overweight individuals often experience these issues due to toxic, fat-producing foods. The lemonade diet addresses skin disorders, infections, cholesterol deposits, and calcium-related diseases, resolving lumps and growths formed as repositories for accumulated waste.

Disease, aging, and death stem from accumulated toxins and congestion throughout the body, leading to crystallization around joints, muscles, and cells. Allopathic medicine's presumption of perfect health until the intrusion of germs or viruses is misleading; instead, defective building materials for cells and organs cause disease.

Growth formations throughout the body act as storage repositories for accumulated wastes. Fungus encapsulates the toxins, trying to dissolve acidic wastes and toxins. Lumps and cysts form as nature's attempt to rid the body of diseases. Cleansing the system halts their development and dissolves them, as these fungi are designed to feed only on inferior tissue when they are starved of acidic wastes.

Nature operates under simple laws where unused materials are recycled or eliminated. Unnatural living accumulates unused materials that manifest as diseases. We often attempt to eradicate them without changing the very behaviors that develop them in the first place and sadly, end up succumbing to them.

The misconception and veiling of these truths have led nations to seek magical cures, resorting to harmful drugs and poisons, further complicating diseases. Simplicity in understanding the body's internal systems and changing one's behaviors to feed the tissues, bones, and blood properly has historically proven the most effective in eradicating negative health conditions.

DR JENSEN PERSPECTIVE ON ALKALINE CLEANSING

Dr. Jensen firmly believed that actively fasting from acid-forming foods while flooding the body with alkalizing tonics, fiber, and electrolytes for proper hydration is a sure method to remove accumulated toxins from the tissues, joints, organs, and fluids of the body, ultimately restoring vitality.

Rest during fasting enhances the body's tone and vitality. Dr. Bernard primarily promoted daily bowel movements as essential for alkalizing. He promoted using pure water enemas or colon hydrotherapy and advised incorporating a laxative at the beginning of alkaline cleansing to prevent autointoxication while addressing chronic conditions.

FUNDAMENTAL PRINCIPLES OF ALKALINE CLEANSING BY CHRISTINE
(Inspired by Dr. Sebi)

"Mucus is the cause of every disease. Eliminate the mucous, and you eliminate the disease." Dr. Sebi

Dr. Sebi's teachings on alkalinity revolve around the body's capacity to easily assimilate substances without imposing stress. Conducting thorough tests on various foods, he meticulously verified their alkaline nature before deeming them suitable for the body's assimilation. Stressing the significance of incorporating as many of these alkaline items as possible into one's diet, Dr. Sebi firmly believed that a more alkaline body leads individuals to a naturally heightened state of consciousness. Conversely, acidity in the body correlates with a lower state of awareness.

Expanding on his research, Dr. Sebi emphasized that diseases flourish in acidic environments, highlighting the inconsistency of employing inorganic substances for disease treatment due to their acidic nature...

He advocated solely for consistently utilizing natural botanical remedies, emphasizing their effectiveness in cleansing and detoxifying a diseased body, ultimately restoring it to its intended alkaline state. Notably, he advised the consumption of items containing seeds exclusively.

Below are a few of these items you can try to implement into your daily regimen. Dr. Sebi recommends only eating items with seeds.

KEY LIMES (SMALL, SEEDED LIMES)

Dr. Sebi recommends squeezing one or two key limes in a glass of spring water as the first drink before brushing your teeth to bring the body into an alkaline state.

RED ONIONS

Dr. Sebi's testing showed red onions were the closest to the original onions that would not cause acid/mucus in the body.

STUDY ON THE INTERACTION OF LEMONS/LIMES WITH WATER.
(Inspired by the Book "Self-Healing Diet" By Brian & Anna Clement at Hippocrates Wellness Center)

A wealth of scientific findings has illuminated the multifaceted benefits of increasing water intake, transcending its role in detoxification. Higher water consumption not only aids in flushing toxins from the body but also serves as a potent tool for regulating appetite facilitating satiety before meals, thereby proving to be an effective weight loss and maintenance strategy.

The pivotal recommendation is to consume approximately 16 ounces of room-temperature water roughly 30 minutes before each meal. However, it's advised not to drink water immediately before or during a meal to avoid potential interference with the digestion process.

A systematic review published in the esteemed American Journal of Clinical Nutrition in 2013 amalgamated findings from 13 studies investigating the impact of increased water intake on weight loss and obesity prevention. The collective evidence gleaned from these studies demonstrated a notable reduction in body weight over 3 to 12 months among participants who increased their water consumption compared to control groups.

Moreover, a study conducted in Germany examined the dietary habits of 1,987 school children. The researchers observed that those who augmented their intake of sugar-containing beverages (such as soft drinks and juices) experienced increased body mass index over a school year.

In contrast, those who opted for increased water consumption did not, demonstrating the preventive role of water consumption in obesity when replacing sugary drinks. To further enhance the fat-burning and preventive properties of water, adding lemon/lime is suggested.

The negative charge and polyphenols in lemons/limes activate water, promoting body detoxification, curbing overeating tendencies, aiding metabolism and digestion, and contributing to weight management.

Additionally, considering the appetite-regulating benefits attributed to ginger (as per Hippocrates), incorporating ginger into water might also be beneficial.

A research study conducted in Korea involved 84 premenopausal women segregated into three groups: a control group without dietary restrictions, a group following a 'placebo' diet, and a lemon juice detox diet group. Following an 11-day assessment period that included measurements of body weight, body mass index, percentage of body fat, and waist-hip ratio, participants in the lemon detox group exhibited positive changes across all evaluated parameters. This data led the researchers to conclude that lemon juice detox reduces body fat, marking it as a potentially valuable component in weight loss regimens.

REFLECTIONS

CHAPTER 3

MODERN INSIGHTS: ALKALINE CLEANSING AND THE GENETIC ROLE OF EYE COLORS
by Cara

"Your genetics load the gun. Your lifestyle pulls the trigger." Mehmet Oz

Enlighten my eyes lest sleep I sleep the sleep of death...Psalm 13:3

The exploration of iris studies boasts a centuries-old legacy, spanning over 6000 years and originating in ancient Mesopotamia. Delving deeply into these studies has yielded profound insights into the importance of the three primary colors of the iris.

This accumulated knowledge is a valuable resource, enhancing our comprehension of how acidic accumulations impact individuals facing many illnesses and diseases. Today, iridology continues to play a pivotal role in advancing our understanding of holistic health on a global scale.

Genetic predispositions influence the body's susceptibility to acids and toxins, leading to inflammation and diseases, often originating from the bowel. Embracing a lifestyle of constant cleansing support incorporating better nutrition, exercise, and stress management is essential for overall well-being. Amid technological exposures, a holistic approach encompassing physical, mental, and spiritual cleansing is advocated.

This transformative journey demands courage, perseverance, and faith, urging individuals to abandon old toxic habits for healthier choices. Though challenging, adopting this nature as a guide reinforces the power of choice for optimal health and happiness. Overcoming fear associated with letting go of familiar yet harmful habits is crucial. Promptly embracing positive changes becomes pivotal in recovering from past mistakes for a happier, healthier life.

A commitment to nature-aligned choices is emphasized, rejecting substances that disrupt the body's balance. Optimal health thrives on whole, natural, and unprocessed elements. Refined sugar, for instance, depletes nutrients, induces acidity, and fuels fungal growth. Remaining open to alternative possibilities prevents intellectual stagnation. If current habits pose risks, seeking knowledge and wisdom in unexplored realms becomes the antidote to a healthier life.

NUTRITIONAL AND CHEMICAL IMBALANCES
(Inspired by Dr. Jensen)

In the intricate web of the body, disruptions, particularly in the form of chemical or nutritional imbalances, also resonate throughout the body, manifesting as illness and disease. Iridology can identify the genetic potential for these subtle imbalances.

Additional health disruptions extend to atomic and electromagnetic levels, where modern technological influences like electromagnetic pollution can disturb natural cellular harmony. Radiation's danger lies in its atomic-level tissue disturbance, breaking down the natural order. Toxic substances infiltrating body tissues, especially in the colon, act as a slow-release poison, eroding vitality and health. Our contemporary environment, laden with toxic chemicals in the air, water, food, skin-care products, and more, has propelled people to unprecedented toxicity levels, contributing to a widespread health crisis worldwide.

Detoxification becomes paramount in this toxic era, aiming to restore balance, peace, and harmony to the genetic health of humankind. Autointoxication, resulting from accumulated chemical and nutritional toxins, impedes wellness. The entire body plunges into a nutritional crisis when the bowel falters, triggering metabolic shock waves throughout every cell and tissue. Beyond the adage "you are what you eat," the essence lies in "you are what you absorb." Even with a wholesome diet, dysfunctional digestive and absorptive processes hinder proper nourishment. Cleansing and nourishing the body with wholesome foods, adequately combined, offers a pathway to healing and disease reversal.

ORGANIC VS. FUNCTIONAL:
(Dr. Jensen perspective)

It is crucial to differentiate between organic and functional conditions. Organic problems necessitate physical interventions, such as altering tissues, rejuvenating cell structures, and optimizing chemical balance. Conversely, addressing functional issues requires a mental shift involving education to promote personal growth, changing attitudes, and embracing a higher path in thoughts, words, and deeds.

While the body is impacted by the mind's choices in adopting a customized approach, encompassing elements like diet, exercise, and cleansing, the organic body accommodates each facet of an individual's distinct needs. Recognizing the influence of belief in exercising willpower through choices reflects a holistic mindset that can lead to enduring balanced well-being.

Uncovering the origins of chronic imbalances involves examining beliefs. Many addictions to food, substances, or behavioral disorders contributing to dis-ease often thrive in the shadows of guilt and shame. Negative choices that persistently harm the physical, mental, or spiritual aspects of overall health serve as manifestations of this pattern. Even if not classified as addictions in our culture, disregarding established boundaries for health care sets the stage for disruptions to reverberate through life.

Below is a brief overview of the three primary iris colors, their indicative characteristics, and general recommendations to foster alkaline balance. These insights empower individuals to make well-informed and health-conscious decisions regarding their holistic well-being.

The information below draws inspiration from Dr. Ellen Jensen's textbook "Techniques of Iris Analysis" and is complemented by Dr. Carol Geeck's client materials from Lifestyle Transformation Health & Research Clinic.

HEMATAGENIC - DARK BROWN
Potential Characteristics:

- Imbalance of blood composition, thick blood
- Inability to store essential minerals.
- Gastrointestinal tract
- Tendency for anemia
- Liver, gallbladder, spleen insufficiencies
- Glandular system, thyroid, adrenal, pineal, pituitary, pancreas

Here is a summary, along with some suggestions to help individuals with brown eyes on their journey to wellness:

Individuals with Hematogenic or dark velvet brown eyes are primarily influenced by the "Hema" or blood system genetically.

The occurrence of blood congestion often results from an accumulation of diverse acids within the circulatory system, exacerbated by poor elimination and liver congestion.

To counter these conditions, it's imperative to steer clear of fried, processed, and junk foods, as well as heated oils, sugar, alcohol, and simple carbohydrates. Embracing a fiber-rich diet through legumes, whole grains, seeds, nuts, fresh sub-acid fruits, leafy greens, and vegetables can significantly prevent various associated illnesses.

Augmenting meals with enzymes aids in enhancing digestion. Additionally, blood cleansing can be achieved through chlorophyll, dandelion root, lecithin, and the consumption of Hibiscus tea with cinnamon. Building a healthier blood composition involves incorporating raw vegetable juices such as beets, black cherries, blackberries, and concord grapes.

Maintaining proper hydration levels, supplemented with electrolytes, is vital for fostering healthy blood.

We strongly advocate alkalizing the body and supporting daily colon and lymph system cleansing. A simple method involves kickstarting the morning with lemon or key lime water, followed by unsweetened celery juice or using a green apple as a natural sweetener.

Consider regular alkaline cleansing, fasting, and periodic detoxification to effectively target liver and spleen health while contributing to overall wellness.

BILIARY- LIGHT BROWN/ MIXED
Potential Characteristics:

- Liver & gallbladder insufficiencies
- Weakness in pancreas function
- Gastrointestinal disturbance and digestive errors
- Disturbances such as constipation, diarrhea, flatulence, blood sugar highs.

Here is a summary, along with some suggestions to help individuals with light brown eyes on their journey to wellness:

Individuals with biliary or mixed eye colors, often called hazel, are governed genetically by the "Bile" system, encompassing the stomach, gallbladder, liver, pancreas, and spleen.

Acidic conditions often contribute to stomach complications, hinder enzyme functionality, and lead to digestive disruptions and blood sugar imbalances.

It is advisable to avoid heated oils, animal fats, and hydrogenated oils. Eliminating or reducing glucose, sugars, honey, maple syrup, and carbohydrates aids in managing blood sugar issues.

The research underscores the significance of limiting and, where feasible, excluding mucus-forming foods—particularly dairy, wheat, sugar, alcohol, caffeine, energy drinks, and drugs—from one's diet. Persistent liver congestion commonly triggers exhaustion, a factor revealed by numerous studies.

Incorporating beneficial oils like cold-pressed olive oil and stable options such as grapeseed, avocado, or coconut oil is essential. Unstable oils become rancid when heated, further burdening the liver. Ensuring green vegetables accompany every meal and choosing lean protein or legumes supports this iris type.

Raw vegetable juices, aloe juice, and lemon or key lime water are recommended to bolster this iris's health. Herbal teas from flaxseed, milk thistle, burdock, or dandelion root can be beneficial. Incorporating chlorella or chlorophyll and moderate amounts of beets supports liver function.

For optimal results, supplementing meals with enzymes, thorough chewing, and adopting a relaxed demeanor during mealtimes significantly benefit this iris type.

Daily colon cleansing, seasonal liver-targeted detoxification, and enzyme therapies have shown remarkable efficacy in fostering ultimate health, as established through extensive studies.

LYMPHATIC- BLUE OR BLUE-GREY
Potential Characteristics:

- Acidic Body
- Arthritic tendencies
- Kidneys need support.
- Allergies
- Fibromyalgia

Here is a summary along with some suggestions to help individuals with blue eyes on their journey to wellness:

The "Lymph" or immune system primarily governs individuals with lymphatic or blue eyes. Accumulations of acidity in lymphatic fluids may trigger hyperactive immune responses, leading to increased mucus and congestion across elimination pathways. Understanding that the lymphatic system oversees the tonsils, adenoids, colon, kidneys, endocrine glands, reproductive organs, lungs, sinuses, and skin is crucial.

To maintain balance, it's advisable to limit or ideally avoid acid or mucus-forming foods such as sugar, dairy, eggs, wheat, simple carbohydrates, red meats, and alcohol. Opt instead for low-sugar, fiber-rich foods and incorporate green foods into your daily diet. Enhance meals with added enzymes.

Celery juice, rich in organic sodium, is recommended for daily consumption. Opt for unsweetened coconut water, sea salt, Celtic or Himalayan salts, and natural electrolytes to ensure proper hydration of lymphatic fluids. Alkalizing these fluids with lemon or key lime water is beneficial. Cleansing the kidneys can be achieved through unsweetened seeded watermelon or pomegranate juice, parsley, oat straw, or horsetail grass tea.

Daily colon cleansing and adequate skincare routines to tone lymphatic channels beneath the skin are vital. Consider incorporating regular fasting and seasonal detoxification targeting the kidneys, colon, and skin to maintain optimal lymphatic health.

ILLUMINATING HEALTH THROUGH IRIS PIGMENTS

Comprehending these iris pigments offers valuable insights into potential genetic health conditions, enabling proactive health management and early intervention.

STRAW YELLOW

Indicates disturbed urinary metabolism, often observed in proximity to the iris wreath.

DARK YELLOW

Suggests long-term inflammation or a low-grade infection. Found at the top of the iris wreath, it may hint at chronic sinus congestion.

ORANGE

Points to potential pancreas or liver disorders.

FLUORESCENT ORANGE

Indicates gallbladder deficiencies.

DARK BROWN PIGMENTS

Associated with liver (hepatic) or pancreatic disturbances.

RUST

Suggests blood sugar disorders or hepatic deficiency.

TRUE RED

Signals potential kidney dysfunction.

TARRY BLACK

This indicates a liver imbalance, potentially indicating a severe overall bodily imbalance.

YELLOW PIGMENTS IN THE WHITES OF THE EYE

Lipid deposits in the sclera (Pinguecula) indicate disturbed fat metabolism. Pterygium is an advanced sclera growth of tissue that may start as a pinguecula.

DISCLAIMER:

This information is not meant for diagnostic purposes but to bring attention to a valuable yet less familiar aspect of iridology within diverse global communities. Its purpose is to offer insights into how this potent tool can be employed to understand and potentially improve health and overall well-being. This approach provides a distinctive perspective on comprehending individual health profiles by exploring the analysis of iris color, strengths, and potential weaknesses. The objective is to illuminate the intricacies of one's constitution, highlighting both inherent strengths and possible weaknesses and illustrating the impact of alkaline cleansing on them.

For those seeking a more profound understanding of how their iris color and its characteristics can reveal valuable insights about their well-being, we encourage you to contact us for a consultation.

We aim to assist individuals on a journey towards heightened self-awareness and informed choices regarding their health. We strongly urge all participants to obtain medical blood work and physical examinations, particularly for those who do not already possess these records. This will empower individuals with valuable health information.

CONTACT THE AUTHORS

For consultations, please email us at
Eye.readologycc@gmail.com

REFLECTIONS

CHAPTER 4

EXPLORING DIGESTION AND ENZYME FUNCTION

*"If you are planning for a year, sow rice.
If you are planning for a decade, plant trees.
If you are planning for a lifetime, educate a person."
-Author Unknown*

A branch from His roots will bear fruit. Isaiah 11:1

ENZYMES AND THE FOUR PHASES OF DIGESTION

This overview of bowel anatomy and physiology aims to acquaint readers with the book's context. While not necessitating expertise, a foundational understanding of bowel basics enriches comprehension. Adhering to principles of right living, the bowel demands awareness and commitment, offering valuable health rewards.

MASTICATION

Digestion of carbohydrates begins in the mouth as saliva is introduced during chewing, breaking down food into smaller pieces that serve as "soil" for the body's roots to absorb nutrients.

ASSIMILATION: THE STOMACH

Hydrochloric acid in the stomach breaks down proteins. Chewing and digestive juices transform food into "chyme," facilitating entry into the small intestine.

ABSORPTION: THE SMALL INTESTINE
"THE ROOTS OF THE HUMAN BODY"

Chyme, entering the duodenum, is highly acidic. Hydrochloric acid and enzymes aid absorption neutralized through bicarbonate in small intestine secretions. Villi are the "roots" that maximize absorption, while fatty products are absorbed through lacteals, connecting with the lymphatic system.

ELIMINATION: THE LARGE INTESTINE OR COLON

Within 8-10 hours, food transitions through the small intestine to the colon. The colon, a reservoir without villi, processes waste and toxins. Chyme becomes semi-solid feces, moved through haustral churning and peristalsis for elimination.

A WELL-FORMED STOOL REFLECTS NOURISHING SOIL FOR STRONG DIGESTIVE ROOTS.

Bacterial activity is minimal in a healthy small intestine, while the large intestine hosts vital bacterial action. The stool's brown color comes from liver-produced bile pigments. A chalky appearance signals bile secretion issues. Taking note of one's stool can receive important biofeedback from the digestive system. Constipation or diarrhea, gas, and strong odors indicate bowel imbalances. Bloating and undigested food in the stool can also be due to poor enzyme function.

DIGESTIVE ENZYMES AND THEIR FUNCTIONS

Digestive enzymes are naturally occurring proteins produced by the body that play a vital role in breaking down food to facilitate digestion. The digestion process involves extracting nutrients from food to fuel your body and enable essential functions. The stomach, small intestine, liver, and pancreas collectively contribute to the production of digestive enzymes. The pancreas serves as the primary contributor to digestion. It generates crucial digestive enzymes responsible for breaking down carbohydrates. Wherein the liver produces bile secreted by the gallbladder to digest fats.

PRIMARY DIGESTIVE ENZYMES

A variety of digestive enzymes exist, and the primary ones are produced in the pancreas.

AMYLASE

- It is produced in the mouth and pancreas and breaks down complex carbohydrates.

LIPASE

- Is produced in the pancreas and dissolves lipids.

PROTEASE

- Is produced in the pancreas and digests proteins.

LACTASE

- Facilitates the breakdown of lactose.

SUCROSE

- Aids the digestion of sucrose.

SYMPTOMS OF DIGESTIVE ENZYME INSUFFICIENCY

Insufficient digestive enzymes can cause discomfort and malnutrition, leading to symptoms like abdominal pain, bloating, cramps, diarrhea, gas, and unexplained weight loss or weight gain. Improve digestion by adding natural enzymes from a health food store to meals and snacks, significantly when health is compromised. Add more enzymes when eating large meals, cooked food, or poorly combined foods. Take enzymes 30 minutes before eating for optimal digestive system preparation.

REFLECTIONS

CHAPTER 5

NUTRITION: ENHANCING ENZYME FUNCTION

"Let food be thy medicine and medicine be thy food."

Hippocrates

I have given you every herb bearing seed, which is upon the face of all the earth and every tree, in which is the fruit of a tree yielding seed. Genesis 1:29

In light of understanding the digestive system and the function of enzymes, choosing the correct combination of foods at each meal to promote bowel health becomes more apparent in an effort to avoid fermentation and indigestion.

GOLDEN RULES OF PROPER FOOD COMBINING
(Inspired by Hippocrates Health Institute)

1. Never eat proteins with starchy carbohydrates in the same meal.
    a. Each group goes well with green vegetables.
    b. Proteins require acid-based enzymes in the stomach to break down properly.

c. Starches use alkaline enzymes in the saliva and the small intestine to digest.
   d. When you put an acid and an alkaline enzyme in the same meal, they neutralize each other and impair digestion.

2. Never eat fruits and vegetables in the same meal.
   a. Fruits and vegetables digest at different rates.
   b. If consumed together, they can cause a backup in the digestive system and produce gas and bloating.

3. Consume only truly ripe fruit when in total health.
   a. Fruit is often picked unripe to extend its shelf life, but if eaten, unripe fruit takes what it needs to ripen from the body.
   b. Fruit contains sugar, and all sugar feeds disease. Sugar is hard on the pancreas, the sugar goes into the bloodstream and feeds disease.
   c. After achieving optimum health, 15% of your diet may be fruit.
   d. When drinking fruit juice, add 75-90% water.

e. Always wash fruit, even organically grown, to remove pesticides and mold.

4. Eat melons alone ~~(with other melons.)~~

   a. Melons digest rapidly and can ferment quickly.

   b. When consumed with slow-digesting foods, they may ferment, leading to discomfort with gas and bloating.

Fig. 2

BAD COMBINATIONS	GOOD COMBINATIONS
Fruit & starch	Protein, sprouts, and vegetables
Fruit & vegetables	Starch, sprouts, and vegetable
Fruit & protein	Avocado and greens
Starch & protein	Avocado and acid or sub-acid fruit
Starch & avocado	Avocados and vegetable
Avocado & protein	

Quick Tip: Pick a starch or protein and add green vegetables. Fruit, eat alone in the morning, starches at lunch, and protein at dinner.

RULES OF EATING
Inspired by Dr. Bernard Jensen

1. Avoid frying foods or using heated oils.
2. Skip a meal if you are not mentally and physically comfortable with the previous one.
3. Only eat when you genuinely crave plain food.
4. Consume food in moderation and avoid overeating.
5. Ensure thorough chewing of every bite. Hippocrates Institute advises chewing 30 times before swallowing.
6. Skip meals during pain, emotional distress, lack of hunger, chilling, or acute illness.

FOOD HEALING LAWS

From "The Health Ranch" in Escondido, California

- Natural food: 50-60% of food should be raw.
- Consume 80% alkaline food and 20% acid food.
- Proportion: 6 vegetables, 2 fruits, 1 starch, and 1 protein daily.
- Vary proteins, starches, vegetables, and fruits from meal to meal.

- Overeating. Overeating can be harmful and potentially fatal.
- Separate starches and proteins. Have fruits for breakfast.
- Cook without water. Cook without high heat. Cook without air touching the food.
- Bake, broil, or roast. If you eat meat, have it lean, no fat, no pork, and eat small portions.
- Use unsprayed, organic vegetables, wash all produce for mold, and eat while they are fresh.
- Use stainless steel, glass, or cast iron for cooking and wooden utensils.

GOOD THOUGHTS, GOOD WORDS, GOOD DEEDS
Dr. Jensen's values

- Embrace decisions, even if not your own.
- Let others make mistakes and learn from them.
- Practice forgiveness and forgetfulness.
- Cultivate gratitude and bless others.
- Seek harmony, even if it means personal sacrifice.
- Avoid discussing illnesses.

- Steer clear of gossip, as it can be toxic.
- Reflect on self-improvement daily, replacing negativity with positivity.
- Incorporate daily skin brushing and use a slant board.
- Consume citrus fruit in sections, not in juice form.
- Limit bread intake, especially with bowel issues.
- Engage in daily exercise, focusing on spinal flexibility, increasing heart rate, and toning abdominal muscles to aid digestion.
- Enjoy grass and sand walks for healthy feet. (also known as grounding.
- Abstain from smoking, excessive alcohol, spitting, cursing, and unclean company.
- Aim for an early bedtime, especially when tired or fatigued.
- Rest more when sick, and consider sleeping outdoors for fresh air.
- Resolve problems in the morning rather than taking them to bed.

THE 80/20 RULE

To achieve optimal health, it is recommended that individuals maintain a diet comprising 20% acid and 80% alkaline-forming foods. Acid-forming foods elicit an acidifying effect, like increased mucus in the body. For example, eating foods that taste acid, like lemon, creates an alkaline reaction, whereas sugar creates an acidic response.

INFLAMMATION AND DIETARY INFLUENCE:

Inflammation, a natural protective response, can arise from infections, injuries, or dietary choices. Scientific evidence supports that sustaining an 80% alkaline and 20% acidic food balance substantially reduces inflammation. Unfortunately, many consume 20-30 times more acidic than alkaline foods. Below are the most common foods.

ACID-FORMING OR MUCUS-FORMING FOODS

- Alcohol
- Sugar
- Coffee, tea, and hot chocolate
- Wheat
- Beef, pork, and chicken
- Dairy
- Eggs

ALKALINE FORMING FOODS

- Fruits: Apricots, apples, bananas, avocados
- Vegetables: Asparagus, broccoli, carrots
- Gluten-free grains: Brown rice and quinoa
- Almonds
- Leafy greens: Lettuce, spinach, kale
- Lemons/Limes

** Studies have found different foods align with varying pH levels on the alkaline/acidic food chart. Ideally, individuals should strive for a diet consisting of 1 acidic food for every 4 alkaline foods consumed. A healthy alkaline-acidic food ratio reduces inflammation, enhances health, and regulates blood sugar, weight, and cholesterol levels.

*** 80/20 can also be a helpful guideline for how much food to eat at a time, encouraging readers to leave 20% of the stomach with room for digestion.

**** Environment will influence diet by providing produce seasonally. In warm climates, raw foods can be obtained easily year-round. In Nordic climates, raw food may be limited. It is recommended to add fermented vegetables like kimchi or sauerkraut.

REFLECTIONS

CHAPTER 6
HYDRATION STANDARDS FOR WELLNESS
Inspired by Dr Sebi

"Nature didn't make any water with chemicals... So, the best water is Spring Water."- Dr. Sebi.

For he shall be as a tree planted by the waters, and that spreadeth out her roots by the river. Jeremiah 17:7-8

Dr. Sebi famously stated, "Water is Life," highlighting its vital role. Water comprises 70% of Earth's surface and 60% of our bodies, revered for its life-sustaining properties across cultures. Its electrified nature allows the absorption of minerals and toxins, making careful water selection crucial.

ENVIRONMENTAL FACTORS

Deforestation and industrial chemicals degrade water quality. Improper storage in metal or plastic containers further compromises its purity. Historical shifts to metal pipes and chemical treatments in water supply systems pose health risks. Different water types have varied impacts. Though chlorinated for safety, tap water eliminates life-sustaining elements and creates harmful by-products. Filters vary in effectiveness and may strip nutrients, while spring water, Dr. Sebi's preference, remains pure and rich in essential minerals.

STORING WATER

In materials like stone, glass, or wood maintain their quality. Purchased bottled spring water might not always meet expected standards, emphasizing the need for vigilance in choosing water sources.

DRINKING A GALLON OF SPRING WATER DAILY

Dr. Sebi advocates and supports optimal hydration and health. Monitoring urine color helps gauge hydration levels. While water remains the best source, other beverages like herbal teas, infused water, coconut water, and broths contribute to fluid intake. Determining daily water intake varies based on age, weight, and climate. The National Academies recommend different averages for men and women. Spring water, rich in minerals and free from additives, aids hydration and bodily functions.

KNOW YOUR WATER SOURCE

Some types of water refine you, and other types degrade you. Learn to discern! Water quality directly impacts health and vitality, making informed choices crucial for optimal well-being. Understanding the qualities of different water types is crucial for overall health. Here's a summary of the current sources of water readily available:

TAP WATER

Chlorination may eliminate waterborne diseases but can create disinfection by-products linked to health issues. It sterilizes the water, removing all life.

FILTERED WATER

Filter reliability varies; some may not remove all contaminants and can eliminate beneficial nutrients, becoming a potential breeding ground for bacteria.

NATURAL SPARKLING MINERAL WATER

Can aid digestion, but be cautious of plastic bottles, as they may contain harmful toxins like BPA. Opt for glass bottles without unwanted additives.

**Beware of CO_2 fizzy or bubbly water. The carbon dioxide can leach minerals from bones.

DISTILLED WATER

Removes impurities but lacks nutritional content. Best used for tea infusions or during cleansing to dissolve calcifications, not as a primary source of hydration.

ALKALINE WATER

(Natural/Man-Made): Natural alkaline water from springs may have curative properties due to essential minerals. Man-made alkaline water varies in quality; nature's version is preferred.

RAINWATER

Abundant and potentially energized if uncontaminated. Dew from morning mist is considered super-energized, especially for plants.

SPRING/GLACIER WATER

Dr. Sebi advocated spring water due to its natural source, neutral pH, and richness in essential minerals. Bottling from your own spring or buying in glass is ideal.

Choosing water wisely involves considering its source and container and avoiding potential toxins from plastic bottles. Each type of water has advantages and potential drawbacks, emphasizing the importance of informed choices for optimal health.

CAUSES OF DEHYDRATION

Every day, your body naturally loses water through activities like sweating, breathing, urination, defecation, and even tears and saliva. Typically, you replenish this loss by consuming fluids and water-containing foods.

Dehydration occurs when you lose excessive water and fail to adequately replace it.

SYMPTOMS OF DEHYDRATION

- Tiredness: Fatigue or feeling unusually tired. Also, insomnia can be expected.
- Dry Skin and Lips: Noticeable dryness of the skin and lips.
- Thirst: Persistent feeling of being thirsty.
- Dark Pee: Urine appears darker than usual.
- Reduced Urination: Not peeing as often as usual.
- Constipation: Not eliminated daily.
- Skin Eruptions: Boils, rashes, or acne.
- Muscle Cramps: Twitching, spasms, and pain.
- Headache: Neck pain and inflammation.

DEHYDRATION TREATMENT:

Maintaining hydration is crucial for overall health, especially during periods of increased fluid loss, illness, pregnancy, or physical activity. Carry a water bottle, ensuring one's drinking enough water throughout the day.

HYDRATION GUIDANCE

One may be dehydrated if experiencing thirst, fatigue, decreased urine output, or signs like muscle cramps, dizziness, yellow or cloudy urine, headaches, or unsteadiness. Drink 4-6 ounces of room temperature water every 30-60 minutes for prime absorption. Ice-cold water is known to disrupt natural enzyme function and inhibit digestion. It is a common practice among health advocates to divide the body weight in half and consume that number in ounces daily to maintain hydration. Example: 150 lbs. ÷ 2 = 75 ounces of pure water daily for maintenance. Consume additional water when cleansing, exercising, sweating, sick or symptomatic, pregnant, or in environmental or stressful conditions.

Replenish body fluids with electrolyte drinks to maintain cellular hydration or to recover from dehydration swiftly.

ENHANCING HYDRATION: NATURAL ELECTROLYTES
by Cara

Vital for a healthy diet, electrolytes like sodium, calcium, potassium, chloride, phosphate, and magnesium found in fruits and veggies offer a preferable organic source over artificial sports drinks, supporting various aspects of well-being. Organic electrolytes are crucial in balancing pH for optimal hydration, aiding nutrient delivery and waste elimination, and contributing to overall cellular support for nerve function and muscle flexibility. Proper electrolyte intake, especially during post-exercise rehydration, helps regulate blood pressure, ensuring stability and promoting overall wellness.

WHAT MAKES SODIUM AN ELECTROLYTE?

Salt is actually a combination of two essential electrolytes — sodium and chloride. These elements are among the list of substances classified as electrolytes. Others include magnesium, potassium, and calcium. The cells use electrolytes to conduct electrical charges to keep your body running efficiently.

Electrolyte ions in the system carry out significant tasks. They help maintain fluid levels, turn nutrients into energy, and support heart rhythm, brain function, and muscle control. Sodium and chloride, the sea salt components, are the body's two most abundant electrolytes. Both are critical in helping cells maintain a proper fluid balance.

Lymphatic fluid, abundant in organic sodium, imparts a salty taste to tears and sweat. Beyond flavor, sodium facilitates nutrient absorption and supports nerve and muscle function, while chloride regulates blood pressure and maintains the body's pH balance.

Sea salt quickly replenishes lost electrolytes, especially sodium, due to sweating. In addition to sodium, it offers magnesium, calcium, and potassium. Choose minimally processed sea salt options like Himalayan or Celtic, found in most grocery stores, and simply add a pinch to water for a convenient and efficient electrolyte boost.

***Table or rock salt is not a source of electrolyte minerals. Use only natural sea salt. ***

BEST SOURCES OF ORGANIC ELECTROLYTES

Organic refers to being derived from nature, not necessarily grown organically. It is bioidentical and easily assimilated by cells, unlike synthetic sources, which may not be optimally absorbed.

COCONUT WATER

Coconut water that is organic and unsweetened is a fresh and nutritious juice derived from palm tree fruits. Served by nature to nurture new trees, it's a vitamin and mineral-rich elixir that naturally replenishes and revitalizes the body. Packed with essential electrolytes such as magnesium, phosphorus, potassium, calcium, and sodium, coconut water rivals the potassium content of a whole banana. Optimal hydration and electrolyte balance contribute to overall well-being. While obtaining coconut water directly from coconuts can be challenging, readily available pre-packaged organic options offer a convenient alternative.

CELERY JUICE

Celery Juice is a potent source of electrolytes, minerals that carry electrical charges. They are crucial in hydrating your body, regulating water balance within cells, and supporting muscle contractions and a balanced pH level. After sweating and exercising, where electrolytes are depleted, Celery Juice is a replenishing and hydrating solution, akin to a sports drink without added sugars and colors.

LEMONS

Lemons reign supreme in the citrus realm for electrolytes, boasting potassium, calcium, and magnesium. Beyond electrolytes, they detoxify the liver, balance pH levels, and fortify the immune system with vitamin C. Enhance any drink by squeezing a whole lemon into warm or cold water for a zesty burst of electrolytes.

WATERMELON JUICE

Watermelon is a hydrating fruit with natural energy, vitamins, and essential electrolytes like magnesium and potassium. Research shows pureed watermelon is as effective as non-organic sports drinks in hydration and energy replacement. It's an excellent organic alternative to sugary sports drinks in your workout routine. Combine watermelon juice with coconut water for a hydrating electrolyte beverage.

BROTH

Soups and broths are rich in electrolytes when sea salt is used to cook. Many vegetables used to make soup are also naturally high in potassium, calcium, and magnesium. Dr. Jensen was an early promoter of using vegetable and bone-based broth to nourish the stomach lining with organic sodium, aiding healthy hydrochloric acid production.

REFLECTIONS

CHAPTER 7

ADDITIONAL STRATEGIES FOR A "NEW START"
by Cara

"The secret to change is to focus all of your energy, not on fighting the old, but on building the new." Socrates.

Forget the former things, do not dwell on the past, see I am doing a new thing, now it springs up Isaiah 43:18

N-UTRITION

Follow the Golden Rules of Proper Food Combining and 80/20 Rules of Eating and add enzymes for balanced nutrition and optimal absorption of vitamins and minerals.

E-XERCISE

Movement is essential every day to assist the lymphatic system in moving fluids through the body. This also stimulates the immune system and builds healthy blood cells. Exercise strengthens connective tissue, muscles, and bones while supporting the nerves and circulatory system. It also improves mental health.

W-ATER

Staying adequately hydrated is vital for health, especially while cleansing. Hydrotherapy practices also use water to help the body remove toxins from the colon, as in enemas or colonics. Bathing and showering can target exfoliation, improve circulation, and promote detoxification through the skin while giving the lymphatic system a massage.

S-UNSHINE

Time outside in nature is vital. 20 minutes of sunshine on the skin promotes vitamin D2 and prevents jaundice. It helps stabilize mental health, reduce inflammation, and promote healthy sleep patterns.

T-EMPERANCE

As defined = The quality of self-restraint, willpower, and self-control. This is a superpower when changing one's health. Become empowered when abstaining from toxic food, drink, substances, people, conversations, TV, and environments.

A-IR

Fresh air and breathing exercises are recommended daily. Oxygen plays a crucial role by facilitating cell replacement, providing energy, bolstering the immune system, and fulfilling other essential bodily functions.

R-EST

Quality sleep is an essential process that enables your body and mind to rejuvenate, ensuring you wake up refreshed and alert. The inadequacy of sleep not only compromises cognitive functions but also poses risks to overall brain health.

T-RUST IN DIVINE POWER

Engaging in prayer, worship, and other spiritual practices can counteract stress responses by amplifying the body's relaxation mechanisms. Faith provides a profound meaning and purpose in life, intricately tied to overall well-being.

COLON HYDROTHERAPY AT HOME
(Hippocrates Guidelines)

ENEMA BENEFITS

Enemas play a crucial role in restoring healthy bowel regularity, especially for those dealing with sluggish or irregular bowels.

Customizable ingredients enhance their effectiveness, like coffee for liver detox or flaxseed tea for inflammation.

ENEMA TYPES:

Cleansing enemas flush the colon gently, aiding conditions like constipation, and is encouraged during cleansing and lifestyle changes to remove accumulated wastes rapidly. The internal use of pure water also massages the internal organs and interior lining of the bowel, stimulating the nervous system, lymphatic vessels, and circulatory system.

Retention enemas, held in the body for 15 minutes or more, stimulate bowel movements and are typically applied to coffee enemas.

ENEMA PREPARATION:

Fasting or special dietary instructions may be helpful before an enema. Ensure sterilized equipment, a lubricant, and purified fresh water at home. To reduce colon pressure, empty the bladder before starting and measure the enema tube to avoid excessive insertion.

AT-HOME ADMINISTRATION:

Enemas can be done at home for cost-effectiveness. Prepare the bathroom to be a healing environment; be sure it is clean, turn on music, read a book, light a candle, and lock the door. This is a time for communion, to pray and release the things that no longer serve the body, soul, and spirit.

STEP BY STEP ENEMA INSTRUCTIONS

1. Spread a towel on the floor, use a pillow for head support, and recline on the right side.
2. Apply lubrication to the tip and gently insert it 2-4 inches into the rectum. Allow the water to flow naturally, filling the abdomen until a sense of fullness is achieved.
3. Clamp the tube, withdraw the tip from the rectum, and then sit on the toilet to release the water naturally.
4. Repeat the process until the expelled water runs clear, ensuring maximum benefits.

RESEARCH ON ENEMAS:

Holistic views support enemas for internal cleansing. Dr. Bernard Jensen advocated for enemas at his Health Ranch, where his patients benefited remarkably. Western medicine employs the use of enemas before and after surgeries.

NATURAL SKINCARE
by Cara

Our skin is our largest organ and is considered the third kidney, as it is also responsible for removing uric acid from the body. Nerve fibers and lymphatic and circulatory vessels lie just beneath the skin. Within 26 seconds, anything on the skin enters the bloodstream and becomes systemic. Read the ingredients of all cleaning supplies and skincare products. It should not be on the skin if it cannot be consumed. Avoid chemical soaps, antiperspirants, lotions, synthetic fragrances, toxic cosmetics, and chemical hair products. Many of these products prevent natural perspiration and are linked to allergies, autoimmune issues, cancer, and hormonal imbalances.

EXFOLIATION

Is important in removing metabolic wastes and environmental toxins from the skin. The gentle massage provided by exfoliation effectively moves lymphatic fluids, breaks up congestion in the tissues, and aids circulation.

SOAKING

In hot or cold water has been used for centuries to treat a multitude of ailments. Bathing is essential for assisting the lymphatic system in removing uric acid from the body. Increasing circulation in hot water invites blood flow to break up congestion in the tissues and skin. Deposits of acids and minerals in the joints, tissues, and organs soften, and painful conditions are reduced.

COLD SHOWERS

Cold plunges invigorate the nerves and lungs while the contracting vessels literally pump the fluids through the lymphatic and circulatory channels. It also contracts the pores of the skin, which is said to reduce aging.

ANCIENT AND MODERN BATHING PRACTICES

Have added minerals, oils, salts, and herbal solutions to bathwater to address specific conditions. Natural beauty has always been illuminated by rigorous soaking, scrubbing, oiling the skin, and herbal skincare.

NATURAL BODY OIL

Opt for natural oils to effectively hydrate your skin. Optimal choices include unrefined, organic, cold-pressed oils. Apply these oils post-shower or bath to nourish your skin, providing a gentle massage to the lymphatic system. This shields your skin from environmental pollutants and imparts a radiant glow to the complexion.

The Essenes, Mayans, Greeks, Egyptians, and various cultures around the world have used bathing as a way to purify the physical vessel to commune with spiritual frequencies. Most temples of antiquity were used as places to heal through prayer and purification practices, using water as the catalyst to remove impurities of both the body and soul.

LYMPHATIC MASSAGE AT HOME

The body is composed of nearly 70% water. Around 8 pints are designated for blood, pumped consistently by the heart throughout the body. However, up to 42 pints of lymphatic fluid primarily circulate through the body due to the movement of the legs and arms. Massage has been used for centuries to promote lymphatic drainage of the vessels and glands residing beneath the skin's surface. The entire lymphatic system gets a thorough massage in the comfort of a private bathroom when regularly exfoliating, bathing, and oiling the skin.

GUIDELINES FOR DRY SKIN BRUSHING

Embrace the rejuvenating ritual of skin brushing, a supreme form of bathing. Unlike soap, it unveils a fresh layer of skin beneath the old cells, renewing itself every 24 hours. The purity of your skin mirrors the cleanliness of your blood.

Skin brushing serves as a catalyst in eliminating uric acid crystals, catarrh, and various body acids. The skin, acting as a powerhouse, is capable of eliminating approximately two pounds of acidic waste daily. This practice also stimulates the lymphatic system, increases circulation, and invigorates the nervous system. For natural beauty purposes, it also activates collagen production, reducing signs of aging, and is effective for breaking up cellulite and lymphatic congestion, assisting in removing unwanted weight in targeted areas.

INSTRUCTIONS FOR DRY SKIN BRUSHING

- Only opt for a natural bristle brush.
- Employ this dry brush each morning before dressing, showering, or bathing.
- Start at the feet and hands, moving toward the heart, brushing in small circles to gently sweep dead skin cells off of the skin.
- Brush the entire body surface, especially the torso, armpits, and thighs, where the lymphatic ducts reside.
- Never brush the nipples.

Consider a softer bristle brush for facial use to complete this invigorating routine.

To address cellulite, it is suggested that grapefruit essential oil be used lightly applied to the bristles of the brush. Place one drop in the palm, rotate the bristles in the oil, and repeat the steps above to target areas of congestion.

Refer to the lymphatic system chart and follow the instructions for lymphatic system massage to promote drainage. Utilize this guide while engaging in activities such as dry skin brushing, exfoliation, or applying oil to the skin.

LYMPHATIC SYSTEM

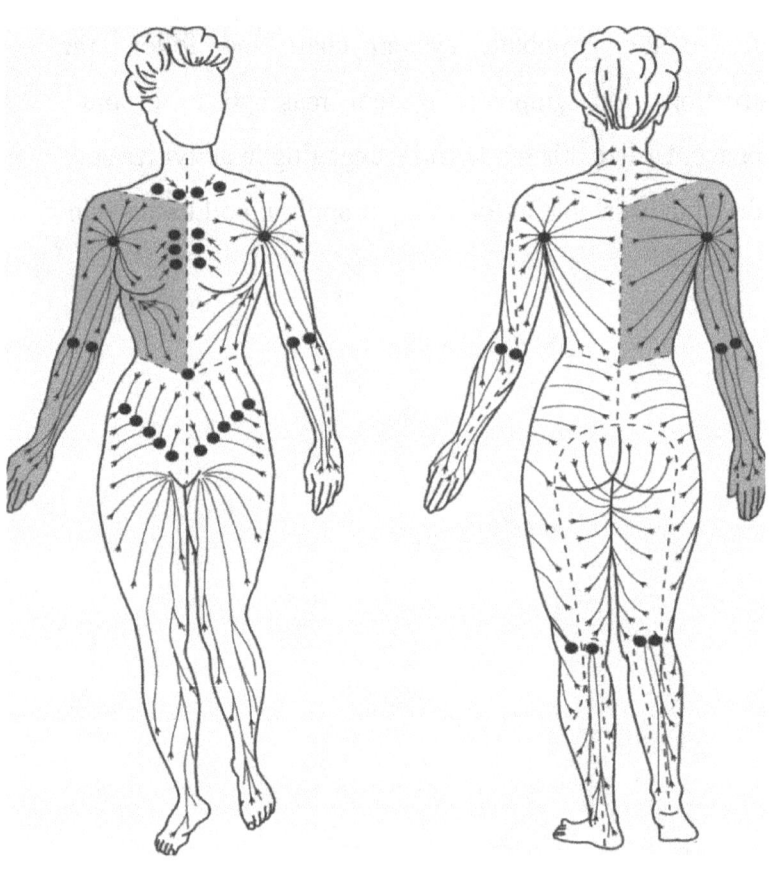

Fig. 3

STEPS FOR AN EXFOLIATING SHOWER

1. Thoroughly moisten the skin with hot water for several minutes to soften the skin.
2. Use a Korean scrub cloth or loofah, with no soap, to scrub the entire surface of the wet skin. Start with the face in small circles. Pay extra attention to the neck, chest, arms, torso, and legs. Noticeable layers of skin are likely to be removed!
3. Now, use natural soap on the cloth and rinse.
4. Pat dry and massage natural oil into damp skin for optimal hydration.
5. Use steam-distilled essential oils as a natural fragrance. Avoid chemicals!!!!
6. Use natural deodorant, makeup, and hair care products. Read labels!!

DETOX BATH INSTRUCTIONS

- Fill the bathtub with warm/hot water and increase the temperature to increase the opportunity to sweat.
- Drink water before and after the bath. Consider drinking ginger tea while soaking to increase circulation and perspiration. This cleanses the lymphatic system.
- Allow at least 20 minutes of soaking time to ensure the completion of the body's cycle for the lymphatic system and blood flow.
- Scrub with a cloth or loofah to increase circulation and exfoliate the skin.
- Pat dry and massage natural oil into damp skin for optimal hydration.
- Use steam-distilled essential oils as a natural fragrance. Avoid chemicals!!!!
- Use natural deodorant, makeup, and hair care products. Read labels!!

Select one of the following products to add to the bath.

Alkalizing Support

1 Pound Box of Baking Soda

Pain Relief + Magnesium To Aide Sleep

½ Bag Epsom Salt

Antiseptic + Cleansing

3 cups Sea Salt

*Increase circulation and perspiration by adding 2 Tablespoons of ginger powder to the bath.

HISTORY AND USES OF ORGANIC CASTOR OIL

Use castor oil for therapeutic purposes. It has a rich history in folk medicine across various cultures. It addresses conditions such as arthritis, liver disorders, muscle spasms, skin issues, and constipation by applying it to areas of congestion and reduced circulation. Castor oil often dissolves fibroids and cysts while benefiting intestinal, liver, and uterine functions when applied as a pack over the abdomen. Additionally, it enhances lymphocytic action, boosts T-cell lymphocyte activity, and balances the autonomic nervous system.

Experiment with the application of organic castor oil by massaging it from head to toe, including the soles of the feet (Be careful of slipping) before bathing or showering to enhance penetration and experience its healing benefits. Use an exfoliating cloth in the water to eliminate dirt and old skin adhering to the oil. Observe the unveiling of hydrated, radiant skin concealed beneath layers of accumulated toxins and old skin.

Castor oil is a deeply penetrating oil that acts as an emollient that removes old skin and reverses aging by deeply nourishing the epidermis. It is considered a beauty aid for use on the eyelashes, eyebrows, and scalp to restore hair growth and help to eliminate dandruff. This oil also addresses cellulite when massaged into areas of congestion.

Castor Oil Pack Materials

- Towel
- Wool flannel or cotton (an old T-shirt works well)
- Saran wrap
- Organic castor oil
- Heating pad or hot water bottle

Instructions

1. Set up a cozy lying space and include a towel to prevent potential oil leakage.
2. Immerse the flannel or cotton in castor oil until thoroughly saturated but not dripping.
3. Apply the oil-soaked fabric to the intended area and wrap it with plastic.
4. Add a small towel and position the heating pad on top, covering yourself to preserve warmth.
5. Unwind for 30-60 minutes, engage in meditation or music listening. Exercise caution with the heating pad.
6. Ensure a continuous and steady application of heat throughout the treatment.

7. Safeguard bedding or clothing from castor oil stains using old towels or plastic.

Reuse

Store the oil-soaked fabric in a sealed container in the refrigerator for recycling purposes. Allow it to return to room temperature before utilizing it again. Please bring it to room temperature before the next use.

Alternate Application

Apply castor oil directly on the skin, cover it with plastic, and follow the heating process, especially for constipation, by massaging the belly in clockwise circles.

When

For non-acute symptoms, use three times a week, alternating days. Once a week or month for maintenance.

Caution

Use caution when using internal castor oil for constipation; it's a strong laxative.

It is not recommended during pregnancy or while heavily bleeding.

REFLECTIONS

CHAPTER 8
SETTING THE STAGE FOR SUCCESS
by Cara

"Do your best and bless the rest." - Hippocrates Health Institute

That person is like a tree planted by streams of water, which yields its fruit in season and whose leaf does not wither – whatever they do prospers. Psalms 1:3

Remember, all great changes come over time. Just for today, do your best. Like gold stars or marbles, consider healthy choices like personal miniature wins to collect daily. Focus on adding healthy choices rather than focusing on removing poor habits.

This is a positive way of reinforcing positive behavior and cultivates wholesome feelings of accomplishment and success versus feelings of failure that often foster rebellious behaviors.

Be realistic about setting daily health goals so they are attainable. It is important to feel good about one's choices at the end of the day to propel the enthusiasm for the next day. Too much internalized criticism is likely to create a rebellion against making lasting change. Be mindful of being kind and forgiving while changing habits. Make a plan the day before, preparing the mind and environment to support the endeavor. Organizing the environment to support the body and mind for the daily self-care that benefits an alkaline lifestyle is encouraged. Setting the stage by cleaning one's personal living space reflects the intention to clean one's internal body as within, so without.

THE KITCHEN

The kitchen is emphasized as a laboratory for experimentation while preparing wholesome food and drinks. Keeping the counters clean creates a sacred space or a living altar for meals to be crafted with intention. The more one prepares food with one's hands, the greater the benefits for body, mind, and soul.

Stocking the kitchen with healthy food is vital to support healthy choices. Exercising substitution assists with making decisions that satisfy the cravings that are likely to arise during the transition from old dietary habits. Having a blender and tea kettle are both very helpful for making many drinks and meals to satisfy the taste buds and flood the cells with nutrition.

Establishing menu plans, writing shopping lists, and experimenting with new recipes can be a fun and creative way of maintaining one's health plan. Also, finding new restaurants or sharing new foods with friends makes eating healthy a delightful experience. Here are some examples.

THE BATHROOM

Create a personal spa in your bathroom by prioritizing cleanliness and a serene atmosphere. Light candles, adjust lighting and use aromatherapy for enhanced ambiance during self-care activities such as listening to music or meditating. Plan ahead for minimal disruptions, especially during increased bowel movements with cleansing. Keep the toilet clean and well-stocked, use a stool for comfort, and organize cleaning supplies. Treat the shower or bathtub as a sacred spa, maintaining cleanliness and considering a water filter. Integrate intention into bathing, focusing on circulation and lymphatic massage. Ensure a spa-like experience with clean towels, body oil, and a robe, leaving you invigorated and ready for the day.

SACRED SPACE

Establishing a dedicated space for contemplation, prayer, and meditation is crucial for integrating emotional and spiritual well-being into an alkaline lifestyle. Choose a quiet location for personal reflection, even within a busy room. Ideally, this space should be separate from the sleeping area or bathroom. Consider creating an altar with meaningful items to reinforce your spiritual connection. During cleansing, uncomfortable feelings may arise as you become aware of subconscious patterns and cravings. Having a designated space to center, ground, and process these emotions is beneficial. Keep a journal to track your physical self-care achievements and document spiritual and emotional growth.

Seeking support from friends or family is encouraged—ask for assistance with chores while prioritizing self-care.

FASTING

"Fasting" in this book refers to eliminating food, substance, or habits that no longer serve the body, mind, or spirit. This can be a potent practice to exercise willpower and build integrity within. It is helpful to start small and work up. It is suggested that one day be designated for self-care, proper nutrition, alkalizing tonics, and meditation with prayer. As one becomes more accustomed to exercising these routines, one day turns into two, then a week, and grows into a lifestyle.

Food is utilized in many traditions worldwide as a religious observance or spiritual development practice. Fasting is common for devotional purposes and has been shown to have significant health benefits. It is important to remember that fasting should not be approached merely as a one-dimensional activity; fasting from certain foods should accompany fasting from specific thoughts, such as worry, anxiety, fear, or anger. Abstaining from vulgar habits is also advised.

Remember to be patient and gradually introduce dietary changes. Fasting should be for a purpose and for a predetermined length of time. As always, remember things that progress gradually take longer to reverse. Patience is a virtue!

THE SCIENCE AND APPLICATION OF PRAYER
by Cara

Let the words of my mouth and the meditation of my heart, be acceptable in thy sight, Oh God. Psalms 19:14

Throughout history, fasting combined with prayer has been recognized as a potent method to cultivate inner strength, resilience and stimulate creativity. This dynamic duo is often employed to prepare the body, mind, and soul for special occasions, rites of passage, or religious celebrations.

Research suggests that, regardless of personal beliefs, engaging in prayer has the potential to alleviate psychological stress. Consistent focus on spiritual values enhances blood flow to the frontal lobes, reduces activity in emotional brain centers, and promotes neurological responses that foster connections and community.

According to Breuning, founder of the Inner Mammal Institute, prayer activates neural pathways, releasing hormones like oxytocin. This impact on serotonin and dopamine neurotransmitters occurs when prayer evokes feelings of love and compassion. The resulting physical and spiritual connection plays a vital role in inhibiting cortisol release, mitigating stress's adverse effects on the immune system, and promoting cellular healing.

Prayer's health benefits include triggering a relaxation response, surrendering control to a higher power, enhancing hope, and evoking positive emotions such as gratitude, empathy, and forgiveness. A study on African Americans with cardiovascular disease suggests that religious practices and spirituality may contribute to improved heart health, often linked to increased self-control for lasting behavioral changes.

For those rooted in spirituality, caring for the physical body as the vessel of the spirit becomes a common ideal. The balanced physical and spiritual union invokes vibrant living, activating one's purpose through exercising integrity—a journey towards becoming a Tree of Life.

A PERSONAL VIEW ON FASTING AND PRAYER/STILLNESS
by Christine

Be still and know that I am God. Psalms 46:10

As a spiritual advisor and certified coach, I've found that combining fasting, prayer, and stillness yields significant benefits, whether for weight loss, health, or deepening one's spiritual connection.

Breathwork is another powerful tool that reduces stress and promotes feelings of openness, love, peace, and clarity while addressing trauma and emotional blocks.

Scientifically proven effects of deep breathing on the heart, brain, digestion, and the immune system highlight its importance. Meditation, or stillness-quietness, calms the mind and body, offering mental health benefits, improved focus, and concentration.

Approaching fasting cautiously consulting a physician is crucial. Committing to a fasting practice, following Habakkuk 2:2 by writing down your vision and entrusting it to God, enhances potential success in any endeavor. In the midst of life's busyness, I termed "LOG" (Life on Go), leveraging tools like prayer, stillness, and gradual fasting transitions is vital. Beginning with liquid meals during specific times and dedicating these moments to stillness can be transformative, echoing Psalms 27:14—waiting on the Lord during fasting and prayer.

Emphasizing the importance of stillness, it's a space for communion with the creator, gaining revelation, and empowerment.

Documenting experiences through journaling is essential, as visions often follow spiritual dreams in this space.

Progressively extending the fasting window, integrating prayer and stillness fortifies benefits. Fasting teaches discipline and surrendering personal will, aligning with the divine will as A Tree of Life, as in Galatians 5:16.

A steadfast commitment to a fasting plan brings immeasurable benefits to the body, soul, and spirit. For guidance or support in initiating a fasting regimen with prayer and stillness, feel free to contact our team for assistance on this transformative journey toward holistic well-being.

BONUS

Unlocking Potential Assistance

Below are the six most common health challenges.
(Inspired by Hippocrates)

DIABETES

Is a chronic health condition that affects how your body turns food into energy. It occurs when your blood glucose, also called blood sugar, is too high. Glucose is a source of energy. The pancreas does not produce enough insulin or cannot effectively use the insulin it produces.

- Diet - rich in green vegetables (raw gives us the most nutrients). Foods cooked at a temperature above 110 destroy the nutrients the body needs.
- Exercise - 30 minutes a day.
- Switch out artificial sugars to low-glucose sweeteners, like monk fruit or stevia.
- Regulate healthy body weight.
- Cleansing - ABC. Cleanse the colon and alkalize.

AVOID:

- Refined Sugar in all forms and saturated fat, starches-carbohydrates.
  (artificial sweeteners)

Tip: Add some "sweet" activities to your life. Make a list of all the things you love to do and do them! Too many people eat sweets because their lives are empty and without joy. Practice generosity, build self-esteem, love yourself, and share happy times with others. Learn to allow and let go. Listen to pleasant music, call a friend, go to a play, take walks in nature. Enjoy the sweetness of life.

Take care of you! It's your life!

CANCER

A disease in which abnormal cells divide uncontrollably, destroy body tissue, and spread to other body parts. It is a disease that results when some cells in our body lose important functions.

- Cleansing is essential. ABC: Cleanse the colon and alkalize.
- A diet high in green RAW/steamed vegetables/Salads, cruciferous veggies, walnuts, berries, beet, garlic, and broccoli. Sprouts are high in antioxidants, helping to fight cancer.
- Remove artificial sweeteners/sugars,
- Starches
- Exercise 30 min a day
- 8 hrs. of sleep is essential.

AVOID:

- Sugars
- Inflammation
- Smoking
- Processed foods.
- Fried food
- Overcooked foods
- Alcohol

HIGH BLOOD PRESSURE/HYPERTENSION

Is the pressure of circulating blood against the walls of blood vessels. A measure of your heart's force to pump blood around your body.

- Regulate and control weight.
- Switch from using table salt to using Celtic or sea salt.
- Exercise
- Eliminate stresses of life
- Eliminate alcohol, coffee, and caffeine-based drinks.
- ABC: Cleanse the colon and alkalize.

ADD:

- More raw vegetables
- Add more fruits (limit if diabetic)
- More water

AVOID:

- Table Salt
- Sugars (Artificial)
- Fried Foods
- Sodas
- Dairy, wheat
- Meats & Fatty foods
- Release Stress
- Caffeine

ARTHRITIS

Is the inflammation of a single or multiple joints. There are many types of arthritis, all of which can be very painful and even incapacitating. An anti-inflammatory diet that helps relieve symptoms is preferred. It is recommended to choose alkaline foods and fast from acidic foods.

- Consume ginger, turmeric, garlic, alfalfa, kelp, and nettle.
- A vegetable and green juice fast.
- Fresh vegetables, especially Asparagus, onions, and leafy greens.

- Some fresh fruits, specifically pineapple, tart red cherries
- Ground flaxseed.
- Avocados
- Foods high in vitamin C
- Natural Black cherry juice (Buy the one that contains no added sugars or preservatives. It is great for breaking up crystals in the joints).
- ABC: Cleanse the colon and alkalize.

AVOID:

- Animal fat, processed fats.
- Nightshades: Peppers, tomatoes, eggplant, white potatoes/bread/starches
- Acidic fruits
- Dairy
- Alcohol

Added relief: Alternate cold gel packs with heating pads. Also, a hot herbal poultice is made up of various dried or fresh herbs, like ginger, and can be beneficial to eliminate pain. Dried herbs, like turmeric, are ground into a paste with a mortar and pestle, adding enough warm water to form a thick paste. The paste is then spread on or between layers of cloth, applied to the skin, and held with a bandage.

**Massage castor oil into the joints or consider using Castor Oil Packs to alleviate pain.

CONSTIPATION

Is the inability to have normal bowel movements. It involves straining, putting great stress on the body. It is even possible to push organs out of place due to the pressure exerted upon them. Certain medications can exacerbate the problem. The solutions are simple and effective.

- Consume - 25-35 grams of fiber daily in the form of fruits, vegetables, and whole grains. Add to the diet slowly over several months.
- ½ your body weight in fluid ounces of green juices, water, and organic herbal teas: The

desire to drink water can dissipate with age. The body will adjust accordingly.
- Suggest prunes & raisins, which are high in fiber, create intestinal contractions and soak up water in the digestive tract, which is necessary for the system to keep moving. Flax water nourishes the bowel.
- ABC: Cleanse the colon and alkalize.

AVOID:

- Alcohol, caffeine, and foods without fiber remove fluids from the body, causing dehydration. Sugar causes fermentation and yeast overgrowth.

SINUS INFECTIONS/ALLERGIES

Are a common recurring problem for many people. A sinus infection is an inflammation of the sinuses and nasal passages. Headaches and pressure in the head area, along with a cough, fever, bad breath, skin conditions, and/or nasal congestion, are common allergy symptoms. They can last for days to many weeks. Raw alkaline foods provide anti-inflammatory effects that can lessen the symptoms over a shorter period.

- Consume - foods high in vitamin C, brightly colored vegetables, freshly made vegetables, and green juices. Steam baths/inhalations with eucalyptus and rosemary essential oils have also been proven to help.
- Flush the sinus with a saline solution.
- ABC: Cleanse the colon and Alkalize.

AVOID:

- Pepper, cinnamon, chili powder.
- Chemicals in cosmetics and cleansing products.
- Exposure to mold or dust.
- Avoid wheat, dairy, sugar, eggs, and red meat.

End Cravings with Spinach, Peppers, & Cinnamon, rich in thylakoids, disrupt craving signals in the brain, proven in studies to relieve unhealthy food urges. As supported by research, Capsaicin from red peppers and EGCG from green tea have documented effects on restraining appetite and controlling cravings.

BENEFITS OF EXERCISE ON BLOOD SUGAR
(Inspired by Hippocrates Health Institute)

In a study published in the prestigious Journal of Sports Medicine, five scientists analyzed seven independent studies focusing on the impact of sitting, standing, and walking on glucose and insulin levels. Participants intermittently engaged in short standing or walking sessions throughout the day for two to five minutes.

The 2022 Sports Medicine publication revealed significant results: Intermittent standing breaks, especially after meals, led to a 9.5% average reduction in glucose levels compared to prolonged sitting. Additionally, intermittent light-intensity walking showed an even more substantial 17% average reduction in glucose levels. Remarkably, just two minutes of walking after a meal had measurable positive effects on blood sugar levels.

This study highlights the crucial role of walking in mitigating spikes in blood sugar levels after meals, occurring typically within 60 to 90 minutes. The beneficial impact stems from walking aiding in the clearance of sugars from the bloodstream, contributing significantly to healthy blood sugar levels, and supporting weight management by using glucose for muscle function.

Furthermore, the study emphasized the profound impact of longer and more vigorous post-meal walks in priming metabolism to burn excess calories. This cumulative effect underscores the long-term benefits of incorporating regular walking routines into daily activities.

REFLECTIONS

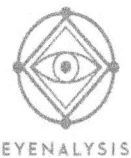

EYENALYSIS

Proper Food Combining Chart

Pick a protien or a starch and pair with green vegetables.
Add oils to starch and vegetable based meals.
Consume enzymes with cooked meals.
Eat fruit alone and in the morning.
Avoid drinking liquids with meals.

PROTIEN	FATS	STARCH
(12 hours)	(12 hours)	(5 hours)
Cheese	Butter	Winter squash
Dairy	Animal fat	Potatoes
Eggs	Nutbutters	Beans
Meat	Oils	Cereal
Nuts		Grains
Olives	GREEN VEGETABLES	Pasta
Peanuts	(5 hours)	Rice
Seeds		Bread
	Asparagus	
	Broccoli	MILD STARCH
	Cabbage	
	Celery	Corn
	Sprouts/lettuce	Peas
	Chard/kale/arugula	Carrots
	Cucumber	Beets
	Garlic/onions	
	Summersquash	

SOUR FRUIT	TART FRUIT	SWEET FRUIT	MELON
(2hours)	(2 hours)	(3 hours)	(2 hours)
Citrus	Berries	Bananas	Honey Dew
Pomegranate	Cherries	Mangos	Watermelon
	Peaches	Grapes	
	Plums	Dates	EAT ALONE
	Apples	Dried fruit	
	Pears		

ONLINE GROCERY RESOURCES

Numerous websites provide information about organic, vegan, and raw food, including suppliers and other resources. For the most up-to-date listings, use a search engine and type in raw food restaurants, living food resources, vegan restaurants, etc.

Door To Door Organics

www.doortodoororganics.com

GreenPeople

www.greenpeople.org

LocalHarvest

www.localharvest.org

Natural Food Network

www.naturalfoodnet.com

Supermarketcoop

www.supermarketcoop.com

Vegdining.com

www.vegdining.com

Vegetarian Resource Group

www.vrg.org

RESOURCES EXPERT

Hippocrates Health Institute
www.hippocratesinstitute.org
800-842-2125

IIPA
www.iridoogyassn.org
205-213-5579
760-736-0291

Bernard Jensen International
www.Bernardjensen.com
760-736-0291

My Infinite Iris
Dr. Ellen Tart-Jensen
www.ellenjensen.com
760-471-9977

SUGGESTED FILMS

NETFLIX
(Excellent teaching tools)

- Healing Cancer from the inside out
- You can heal your life.
- Forks over knives
- Escape the fire.
- Human: The World Within
- Poisoned: The Dirty Truth About Your Food
- You Are What You Eat

REFERENCES

LifeForce – Brian Clement, Hippocrates

The Electrical Body vs Weightology – Christine Maxwell

Self-Healing Diet – Brian Clement, Hippocrates

Techniques in Iris Analysis – Dr Ellen Tart Jensen

Health is your Birthright – Ellen Tart Jensen

Cara

The Essene Gospel of Peace - Edmond Bordeaux Szekely

Tissue Cleansing Through Bowel Management - Dr. Bernard Jensen

Master Cleanser - Stanley Burroughs

The Alkalizing Diet - Istvan Fazekas

Proper Food Combining - Lee DuBelle

Clinical Handouts- Lifestyle Transformation Health & Research Clinic

Return to Eden – Jethro Kloss

Heal ThySelf – Queen Afua

AFFIRMATIONS/PRAYERS

Cara and Christine have seamlessly integrated the powerful practice of incorporating prayers and affirmations into their daily routines, recognizing the profound impact of infusing positivity and life-affirming statements into their daily lives. This intentional habit has become a cornerstone of their existence, extending its influence on their educational pursuits.

By prioritizing the spoken manifestation of positive thoughts and affirmations, they enrich their lives and contribute to a more uplifting and encouraging environment for those around them. This mindful approach to daily living transcends individual growth, presenting potential benefits that resonate with the broader community.

Through their commitment to fostering a positive mindset, Cara and Christine exemplify the transformative power of incorporating spiritual and affirmational practices into the fabric of everyday life.

PRAYER

Holy, Eternal Loving Presence (HELP), I present myself to You, body, soul, and spirit. Guide me today as I seek to live in my God created purpose and will. I need you in all that I do. Direct my path, order my steps in your divine will for my life. Be a lamp unto my steps and a light on my path. Grant me sweatless success in everything I set my hand to do that aligns with Your purpose for my life.

I thank you and give you all glory, honor, and praise. Amen/selah.

Christine

SUPPLICATION

I call upon the Creator of all that is past, present, and eternal. With gratitude overflowing in my heart, I come to you today.

I humbly request liberation from all things that no longer serve me and create dis-ease.

May balance be restored in every facet of my being - physical, spiritual, emotional, mental, and financial. Grant me the gift of wisdom to illuminate my path. Guide my every step and provide me the resolution to select sustenance for my body, mind, and soul in harmony with the divine purpose for my life. Deliver me from temptation and restore my soul. I thank you for making all things possible for those who believe. As for me and my body temple, I serve the Most High plan for my life and create a sanctuary for my soul to reside in my body. Amen

Cara

AFFIRMATIONS

Cultivate profound inner harmony by engaging in the transformative "I am" exercise, a powerful tool to restore balance and foster a sense of equilibrium in your life.

> I am healed
> I live in my Divine DNA
> I am an overcomer
> I am confident
> I am whole
> I am loved
> I am bold
> I am free
> I am prosperous.
> I am brave
> ## I AM A TREE OF LIFE

CONTACT THE AUTHORS

For consultations, please email us at
Eye.readologycc@gmail.com

Christine Maxwell

Iridologist
Certified Health Educator
Certified Alkaline Wellness Coach
Ordained Minister
www.KingdomResourceCenter.us

www.iridologyeyenalysis.com
christinemaxwellcplc@gmail.com

(954) 271-1174
(770) 800-3309

Cara Marie Ringland

Iridologist
Traditional Naturopath
Detoxification Consultant
Registered Thai Massage Instructor
www.bodytemplehealth.com
iris.eyenalysis@gmail.com
(530) 263-2125
(770) 800-3309

www.ingramcontent.com/pod-product-compliance
Lightning Source LLC
Chambersburg PA
CBHW072031170426
43200CB00025B/2478